616.
RiV

PAIN

PAIN
FROM SUFFERING
TO FEELING BETTER

Marie-Josée Rivard Ph. D.
with Denis Gingras Ph. D.
Foreword by Yoram Shir
Translated by Barbara Sandilands

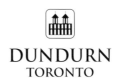

DUNDURN
TORONTO

Editor: Michael Melgaard
Design: Courtney Horner
Printer: Marquis

Library and Archives Canada Cataloguing in Publication

Rivard, Marie-Josée
          [Douleur. English. 2012]
     Pain : from suffering to feeling good / Marie-Josée Rivard ; with Denis
Gingras ; foreword by Yoram Shir ; translated by Barbara Sandilands.

Translation of: La douleur : de la souffrance au mieux-être.
Includes bibliographical references.
Issued in print and electronic formats.
ISBN 978-1-4597-2351-1

1. Pain--Popular works. 2. Pain--Treatment--Popular works. 3. Pain--
Psychological aspects. I. Gingras, Denis, 1965-, author II. Sandilands,
Barbara, translator III. Title. IV. Title: Douleur. English. 2012.

RB127.R5813 2015   616'.0472   C2014-907102-7
                                                               C2014-907103-5

          1   2   3   4   5   19   18   17   16   15

  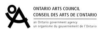

We acknowledge the support of the **Canada Council for the Arts** and the **Ontario Arts Council** for our publishing
program. We also acknowledge the financial support of the **Government of Canada** through the **Canada Book Fund**
and **Livres Canada Books**, and the **Government of Ontario** through the **Ontario Book Publishing Tax Credit** and the
Ontario Media Development Corporation.

Printed and bound in Canada.

Visit us at
Dundurn.com | @dundurnpress | Facebook.com/dundurnpress | Pinterest.com/Dundurnpress

Dundurn
3 Church Street, Suite 500
Toronto, Ontario, Canada
M5E 1M2

To the women and men with chronic pain I've met over the years, who've shared their stories and given me the privilege of understanding what they were going through. Your perseverance and your search for wellness are a constant source of inspiration. This book is for you.

Table of Contents

Foreword

BY YORAM SHIR, MD

Humans differ substantially from one to the other. We differ in our sex and ethnic origin, in the conditions and climate in which we live, in the food we consume, in our genetic heritage, and in our diverse life experiences. Nevertheless, there are things common to us all, one of the most obvious of which is the perception of pain. From the day we are born until the day we die, we all experience pain almost daily. Pain of diverse origins has become so embedded in our lives that its mere existence is perceived as almost normal and, many times, as an acceptable phenomenon. Painful perceptions such as an occasional headache, a muscle ache ensuing from physical activity, abdominal pain, minor incidental injuries, and pains associated with menstruation, to name just a few, are familiar. In most cases, this familiarity is reassuring, since past experiences have taught us that these types of pain tend to resolve and disappear quickly. Even when we experience major trauma, injury, or surgery, events that could be associated with severe pain, the natural course of healing is often a gradual reduction in pain until its disappearance.

Our perception of incidental acute pain, even when severe, as a temporary symptom makes it difficult, and sometimes impossible, to comprehend and accept the fact that pain can actually become a chronic disease in its own right. A disease that in many respects is similar to other common chronic ailments such as ischemic heart disease, hypertension, and diabetes. The difficulty of accepting chronic pain as a disease is not the domain of pain sufferers alone. Others, including their loved ones, society in general, and, many times, the medical community itself, share the same difficulties. How else can we explain the fact that chronic pain — one of the most common ailments known to humankind, affecting at least 20 percent of the world's population — is so underestimated and undertreated?

Our inability to fully understand chronic pain and its effects augments the suffering of people affected by it beyond the burden of the disease itself. Take for example a patient with long-standing insulin-dependent diabetes who needs careful and constant control of his blood sugar. Try to imagine his emotional response (not to mention the medical consequences) if exposed to comments like: "Get a hold of yourself," "Stop complaining and go on with your life," and "You don't need all these medications you insist on taking." This kind of attitude, unlikely to appear when coping with the diabetes itself, might surface when coping with painful peripheral neuropathy — one of the most devastating consequences of diabetes, characterized by an intractable and constant burning pain in both feet. While the feet maintain their normal appearance, this pain could prevent patients from walking properly, wearing shoes, or even covering their feet with a sheet when lying in bed at night. Can we really understand and accept such pain-mediated complaints? No wonder that many of those afflicted by chronic pain prefer to suffer in silence once they realize that others cannot comprehend the meaning of living with chronic pain.

My clinical practice, spanning more than two decades, has mainly been dedicated to the treatment of patients with chronic pain. During these years our understanding of basic pain mechanisms has increased significantly. More importantly, there are at last signs that the public, the medical community and governments have all become more attuned to the disease and its devastating consequences.

It has become clearer that chronic pain is a multi-faceted disease involving both body and mind, and that for many patients a single intervention will not suffice. Nevertheless, chronic pain is far from being conquered, and our ability to cure, and even to properly treat patients suffering from it, is still limited. Our limited abilities are frustrating not only for patients. We, the clinicians, are almost equally frustrated because of the growing gap between the substantial scientific advancements in chronic pain research and our limited capacity to heal it. Like many others, I therefore strongly believe that the first step in trying to overcome the epidemic of chronic pain is to raise awareness of the problem and to enhance chronic pain education among the public and the medical community. In this context, *Pain: From Suffering to Feeling Better* is a timely and much-needed addition to the literature on chronic pain. This book is based on the extensive experience of the author as a clinical psychologist attending to, and treating patients with, chronic pain in a multi-disciplinary pain centre. It explores such topics as the basic mechanisms of the phenomenon of pain, its vast effect on patients' well-being, the critical importance of the equilibrium between body and mind, common therapeutic options, and the importance of self-healing approaches. Hopefully, it will contribute to the ongoing efforts to win the battle against chronic pain.

Yoram Shir, MD

DIRECTOR
ALAN EDWARDS PAIN MANAGEMENT UNIT
MCGILL UNIVERSITY HEALTH CENTRE
MONTREAL

Foreword

BY GUY CARBONNEAU

In my career as a hockey player, I was used to living with pain, caused by the hits and injuries I experienced, as well as the constant physical demands placed on my body in every game, both in the regular season and in the playoffs.

At around 36, I started to feel pain in the groin, a pain different from all the others. I tried, like I always had, to adapt my fitness training to deal with the pain, but the more I trained, the more it hurt. The pain became more and more intense and worrying, until the day when, after several medical consultations, I got the verdict: early osteoarthritis in the hip. I wasn't even forty yet.

My doctors told me I couldn't have my hips operated on because I was too young, that I'd have to wait until I was sixty-five and that I'd have to learn to live with the pain. I wondered how on earth I could stand this pain for the next twenty-five years. I would have a lot of pain for a month and then go for three or four months without pain. As the years went by, the periods without pain became less and less frequent until the pain became constant.

I didn't believe it was "normal" to have pain every day. I very soon had to stop skating, and even when I was coaching I couldn't skate with the players. I had to stop running and had more and more trouble playing golf, because walking had become difficult and painful. I tried to adapt my training by taking up cycling, which I managed to do and which meant I could keep in shape. Not only were my sports activities severely put to the test, my nights were also very difficult: I couldn't find a comfortable position for getting to sleep or figure out which side to sleep on, because my hips caused me pain. My sleep was interrupted and sometimes I was impatient and irritable the next day. I wondered what the future held for me.

In 2009 I was able to take advantage of new technology and underwent a double hip replacement; this gave me back my mobility and — most importantly — meant I was once again pain- free.

Today I'm no longer in pain. I'm aware of how difficult the years spent in pain were. Luckily, I had several training techniques I used to help myself as much as possible. I had understood right from my early days in hockey that I was responsible for my body and that I constantly had to adapt my activities to my physical condition, whether it was a shoulder injury or chronic pain. All during this period, I held onto the hope that one day a treatment would relieve my pain. I channeled my energies into the positive aspects of my life, kept my spirits up as much as possible and tried to avoid making my family and friends suffer the consequences of what I was going through. I stayed active, concentrating on what I could do, instead of on what I couldn't.

I've now resumed a life I had lost for several years and I'm making the most of it. I've met many people with chronic pain and I understand only too well what they are going through. I often tell them that to feel better you have to help yourself, not shut yourself away alone with your problem, and — despite the pain — do everything you can to be sure you get the most out of life.

Guy Carbonneau
ATHLETE, FORMER PROFESSIONAL
HOCKEY PLAYER AND COACH

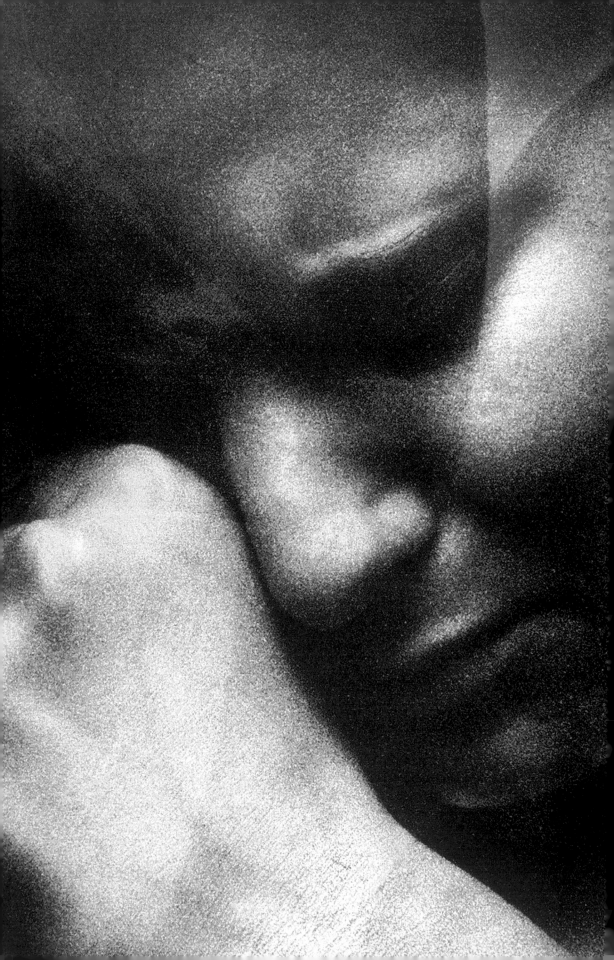

Introduction

From birth to death, we all have to deal with a series of painful events that will have a profound influence on our personality and perception of the world. Difficult challenges, whether they entail mourning for our loved ones, romantic, family-related, or professional setbacks, or illnesses and serious injuries, can present themselves at any time and have an impact on our lives, from a physical as well as a psychological point of view. Death may be the inevitable outcome of life, but the fight against pain and the search for well-being are its central themes, inextricably linked to the human condition.

Most of the time, these challenges can be overcome by human beings' incredible adaptability, our innate capacity to mobilize our emotional and physical resources to cope with adversity, and, in one way or another, learn once more how to live more or less normally after a serious physical injury or a painful emotional event. This fundamental trait of the human soul is especially well illustrated by the resilience of people who have survived dreadful situations that have devastated their lives and those of their loved ones (wars, genocides, natural disasters) or by the courage shown by those who have to deal with intense emotional hardships like the death of a child or trauma caused by abuse.

Needless to say, this innate ability to adapt to pain, in particular pain related to physical trauma, depends largely on how intense the pain is and, most importantly, on how long it lasts. Anyone who has had a serious accident, undergone an operation on particularly sensitive vital organs, or been struck by sudden pain (appendicitis, a kidney stone) knows how difficult it is to tolerate acute pain. Fortunately, thanks to remarkable advances in modern

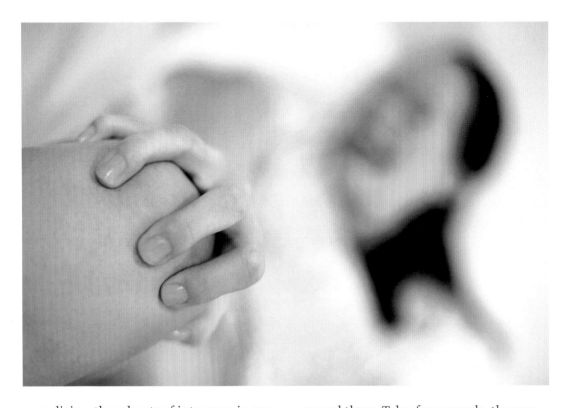

medicine, these bouts of intense pain are often temporary and diminish gradually as the injury heals or the source of the discomfort is removed. As a result, even though the potentially lethal dangers associated with such acute pain can give those affected the "fright of their lives" and have a permanent impact on their perception of the fragility of life, the fact that it doesn't last long makes it easier to manage and accept.

However, the situation is very different when the pain persists for long periods and becomes chronic. As great as our innate capacity to handle temporary pain is, this ability is poorly adapted to constant pain affecting every aspect of daily life. Constant pain, combined with a deterioration in physical ability, is very hard for sufferers to accept, as it dramatically changes the way they interact with those around them. Take, for example, the case of a formerly active and athletic young woman who, following an unfortunate workplace accident, has been living with constant pain in her arm and shoulder, which considerably limits her movements and activities. Or that of a young father with chronic backache, for whom playing ball with his children is now just a memory from the past when he didn't have pain. And what about the elderly person who can no longer sleep well, because just the sensation of lying on a mattress is painful, or patients with diabetes whose difficulty in coming to terms with the pain in their legs is only matched by the fear of seeing their health deteriorate and having to undergo an amputation. Living with chronic pain can become an unending torture that can completely ruin a life if it's not managed well.

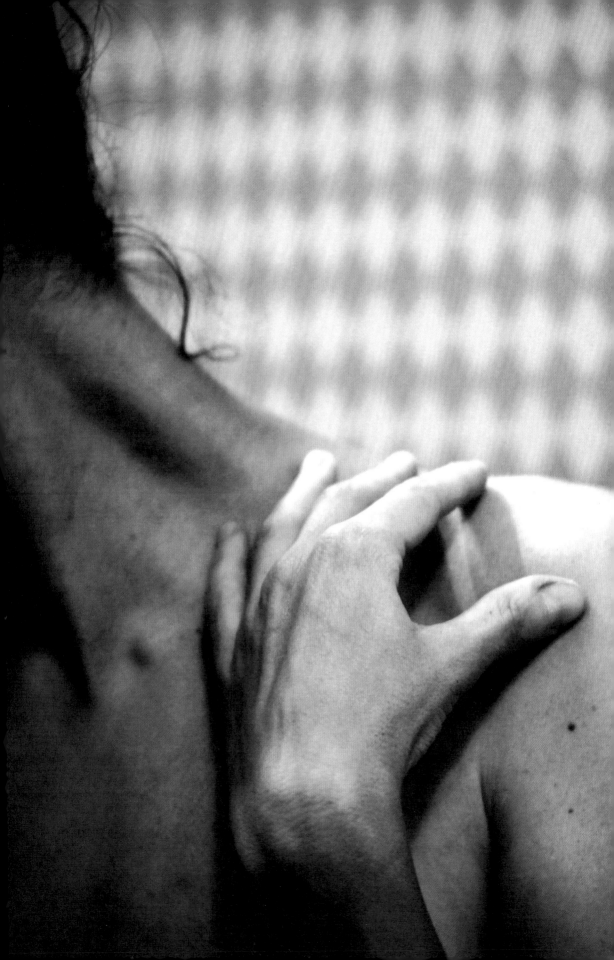

The physical impact of chronic pain obviously has a number of repercussions on the morale of those suffering from it. Anxiety, anger, depression, despair, and even suicidal thoughts are frequent phenomena in people with chronic pain, and this psychological suffering tends to make the effects of the physical pain worse. In situations like these, chronic pain doesn't just affect our ability to work, carry out everyday tasks, or take part in our usual leisure activities — it also influences our moods, our personality, the very essence of what defines us as individuals. This kind of physical and psychological pain is even harder to manage because of its private, intimate nature, which makes it hard to communicate clearly and precisely to medical personnel and friends and family. Feeling like their pain is holding them prisoner and that they are being left on their own, people with chronic pain may thus find themselves drawn into a vicious circle, where pain takes hold of every aspect of their lives, isolating them more and more from the outside world.

This kind of situation is, however, far from inevitable: many scientific studies have shown beyond a doubt that it's possible to adapt to chronic pain and weaken its grip on the lives of people living with it. Pain is not just an unpleasant sensation resulting from physical injury; on the contrary, it's an extremely complex process involving a number of physiological, genetic, hormonal, and emotional factors that together have a determining influence on how we experience pain. This combination of physiological and psychological factors means that the effective treatment of chronic pain requires not just a therapeutic approach involving drugs and physical medical interventions, but also a psychological approach that targets the emotions involved in pain perception.

In this perspective, we felt it would be useful to provide an overview of the current state of scientific knowledge about chronic pain and its impacts on day-to-day life and morale, as well as the medical and psychological therapeutic approaches that are effective in managing it and can be applied to everyday life. Using clinical examples illustrating the main kinds of chronic pain experienced in the population and the emotions people in pain have to cope with, we suggest ways to help you better understand the public health problem that pain represents, a problem for which we simply must find solutions to improve the sufferers' quality of life.

We must not remain passive in the face of chronic pain, nor accept with resignation the burden it places on our lives. But to overcome this challenge, we must first of all become "the expert" on our pain; we must be the best informed about our own condition, the possibilities and limits of the medications we are taking, and the need to better manage the emotions the pain causes. By gaining control over what chronic pain really is, we can begin to develop our inherent ability to adapt to it. We can approach it in a more positive way and develop a constructive "anti-pain" approach calling on a broad range of therapeutic options by taking aim at both its physical and psychological aspects. Even if we can't entirely eliminate chronic pain, it is nonetheless possible to adapt to it and stop it from taking centre stage in our lives.

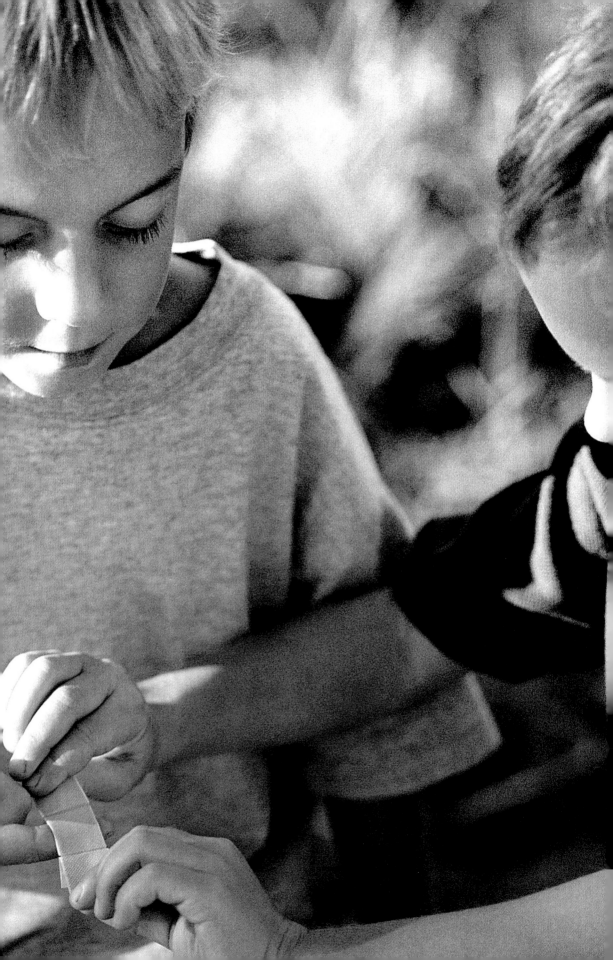

CHAPTER 1

The Problem of Pain

"I think, therefore I am" is the statement of an intellectual who underrates toothaches. "I feel, therefore I am" is a truth much more universally valid, and it applies to everything that's alive.

— MILAN KUNDERA

The acquisition of language is a fascinating stage in child development, as it reflects in a tangible way children's awakening to the world around them, as well as their desire to become part of it by expressing their thoughts and emotions. It is remarkable that in every language's childish vocabulary, the first words used to designate the key elements of daily life in early childhood, such as the most important people (mommy, daddy) and certain situations (beddy-bye, pee-pee), also include the unpleasant feeling associated with a painful situation. Whether it be *bo-bo* in French or Russian, *booboo* in English, *bua* in Italian, *pupa* in Spanish, *buba* in Serbo-Croatian or *kuku* in Polish, to give just a few examples, all of these childhood words indicate the fundamental place that pain holds in our lives from very early on and our innate impulse to express its influence in a concrete way.

Whether small or big, these childhood booboos are usually acute forms of pain, which means that although they occur suddenly their unpleasant effect subsides quickly, owing to good care from parents or, in the case of more serious injuries, from medical professionals. These first encounters with pain are very important, not only for learning to avoid dangerous situations, but also because they have a lasting influence on the way we view pain throughout our lives — as an upsetting but temporary event. As our parents often told us, "It'll be over soon!" Achievements in modern medicine mean that we have actually acquired the ability to fight the acute pain caused by a number of serious kinds of trauma, such as fractures, injuries resulting from work, or traffic accidents, as well as very painful and potentially deadly inflammation, like appendicitis or pancreatitis. Without a doubt, these advances are among the medical contributions that have had the greatest effect on improving people's living conditions; their effect has been such that for most people, the word "pain" mainly refers to acute pain, something that certainly does have an effect on us, but is nonetheless temporary.

PERSISTENT PAIN

Bouts of acute pain are part of our lives right from birth and act like warning signals to protect the body from threats to its well-being. And in the course of a lifetime, there are certainly no lack of dangerous situations! Cuts, burns, various kinds of shock, operations, serious illnesses — all of these onslaughts are detected by our body's network of sensory nerves and are immediately relayed to the brain to let it know something dangerous is present. This pain sensation, called nociception — from the Latin *noceo* (to harm) — doesn't usually last very long, but can sometimes be extremely intense, reaching the limit of human endurance.

However, acute pain from a specific injury or wound is just one of many painful situations we may have to face during our lifetime. In some cases, acute pain recurs over long periods and becomes a chronic and persistent problem from which sufferers get very little respite (Figure 1). For example, postoperative trauma, diabetic neuropathy, and post-herpetic neuralgia (shingles) all cause intense pain that often responds only partially to analgesics and remains very difficult to treat. These kinds of chronic pain run counter to our usual perception of the phenomenon of pain; they have unique characteristics that give them a dimension far greater than the temporary unpleasant sensation typical of acute pain.

In addition to the fact it lasts longer (more than three months, sometimes several decades), chronic pain can manifest itself in three ways. For many people, the physical trauma causing the pain (surgery, injury, illness) is well documented and provides an explanation for the pain's intensity; treatment, however, has very little effect. In

THE MAIN DIFFERENCE BETWEEN ACUTE AND CHRONIC PAIN

	Acute Pain	Chronic Pain
DURATION	3 to 6 months or less	more than 3 to 6 months
SOURCE	known	• known but more or less resistant to treatment • unknown
FUNCTION	useful and protective (warning signal of an injury)	useless and destructive (false alarm)
THERAPEUTIC GOALS	permanent eradication through treatment (drugs, surgery)	relief, better pain management and enhanced quality of life

FIGURE 1

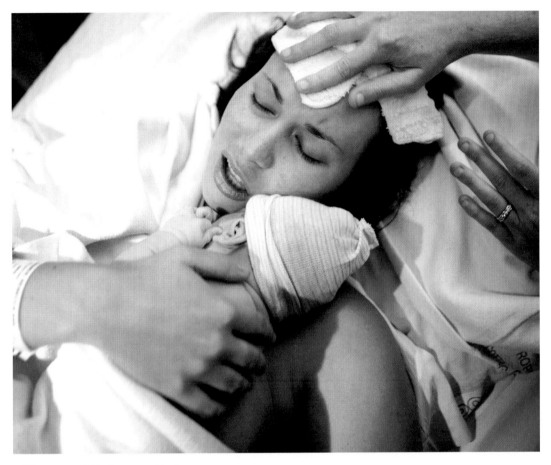

Types of Extreme Pain

Childbirth

Giving birth to a child involves one of the most intense kinds of acute pain, according to the pain index developed by Dr. Ronald Melzack of Montreal's McGill University. The mechanisms that cause this pain are different in the two phases of labour. During the first phase, the pain is essentially due to uterine contractions, as well as the dilation and stretching of the cervix. The pain felt as the baby is expelled from the uterus is caused by the distension of the pelvigenital canal (the birth canal) and the muscles of the pelvic floor, which are connected to the spinal cord by several nerves. It's medically possible to reduce the pain by blocking the sensation transmitted by these nerves using an epidural anaesthetic, a procedure in which an analgesic is injected close to the membrane surrounding and protecting the spinal cord (the dura mater). But despite its intensity and the physical challenge it represents, the pain of childbirth is different. It's "positive" pain, since it's one of the rare kinds of intense pain associated with a happy event: the birth of a child.

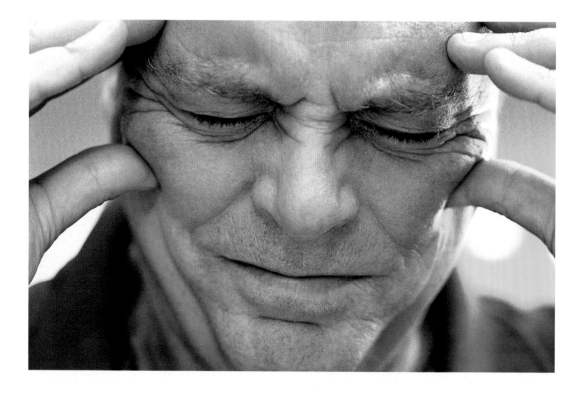

Renal Colic

Usually caused by kidney stones that block the flow of urine, renal colic is an extremely intense pain in the lower back that radiates outward to the genital organs. It occurs more often in men and strikes suddenly, causing great discomfort, since finding a position to alleviate it is impossible. Some people experience chronic renal colic at regular intervals; this is a very debilitating condition that can, over time, interfere with kidney function. Luckily, even though most stones pass on their own without medical intervention, the development of ultrasound technology (extracorporeal lithotripsy) has improved treatment in the most difficult cases. Ultrasound pulverizes the stones through the skin, without invasive procedures, so they can be eliminated naturally.

Cluster Headaches

Considered to be one of the worst kinds of pain a human being can experience, this headache is caused by a dilation of the blood vessels and an inflammation of the branches of the trigeminal nerve behind the eye. This inflammation causes intense pain usually accompanied by a drooping eyelid (ptosis) and excessive watering of the eye. The pain radiates toward the forehead, jaw, or other parts of the head, usually on the same side, and reaches its peak about fifteen minutes after the onset of symptoms. This pain has earned cluster headaches the nickname "suicide headache," as people who get them may feel desperate and try any means to be rid of them.

other cases, a trauma, well documented or not, doesn't explain the intensity of the perceived pain, nor the subsequent disability. Lastly, for still other people, the pain persists in the absence of specific injuries, or even long after they've healed: it's actually not uncommon for people to suffer very disabling chronic pain, even when medical examinations reveal nothing abnormal. Obviously, this is an extremely frustrating situation, for both doctor and patient, as being unable to explain the causes of the pain deprives us of a vital point of reference to make managing it easier. Pain that lasts, with or without apparent reason, is troubling and can impose a heavy physical and psychological burden.

The acute and chronic forms therefore represent two very different aspects of the pain phenomenon, both from the viewpoint of the mechanisms at work and in terms of their impact on the quality of life of sufferers. Acute pain may be considered a beneficial phenomenon, a kind of "pain-alarm" designed to protect the body from the danger caused by an injury, for example; chronic pain, on the other hand, is a "pain-illness," a pathological state in which the body's alarm system is completely out of control and becomes instead a destructive force for the sufferer. This is because persistent pain is not restricted to just one part of the human body: the entire individual is affected, with all the physical and psychological repercussions this entails.

A LARGE-SCALE PROBLEM

In Canada, as in all industrialized countries, it's estimated that roughly 20 percent of the population suffers from chronic pain; in up to one-quarter of these people, the pain can be so intense that it imposes limits on most normal activities (Schopflocher et al., 2011; Boulanger et al., 2007). This is a public health problem of considerable scope,

THE MAIN CHRONIC CONDITIONS OCCURRING IN THE CANADIAN POPULATION

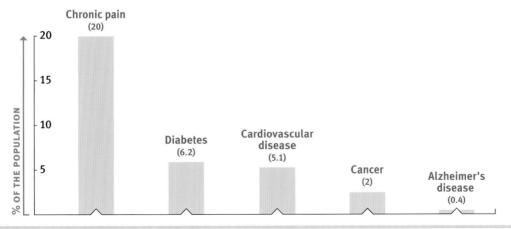

FIGURE 2   Reitsma et al., 2011; Statistics Canada, 2007–2008

affecting more people than cancer, heart disease, diabetes, and Alzheimer's disease combined (Figure 2).

Like most chronic illnesses, pain occurs predominantly in the elderly, with the burden falling particularly heavily on women: 21 percent of men and 31 percent of women over sixty-five suffer from chronic pain, with these percentages rising to nearly 40 percent among seniors living in health care facilities (Figure 3). However, chronic pain is not exclusively associated with aging and it can even be considered a relatively frequent phenomenon among younger people. For example, approximately one Canadian in ten under the age of forty-five is dealing with chronic pain — no fewer than two million people (Ramage-Morin and Gilmour, 2010).

Despite its high prevalence, chronic pain nonetheless remains a "silent" illness, very seldom discussed in the media, whose impact is still underestimated to a great degree. This paradoxical situation can largely be explained by the veil of mystery surrounding anything to do with pain, and in particular the great difficulty we have in precisely describing the extent of its effects on the human body. In contrast to the main illnesses that affect people, which can be diagnosed using an impressive arsenal of sophisticated machines or ultra-sensitive blood tests, there is no "detector" that can "measure" pain, or precisely quantify its intensity as perceived by the sufferer. More than any other health problem, pain is a personal and subjective experience, with the burden it entails remaining invisible from the outside. Chronic pain is thus a truly silent tragedy, a condition whose devastating effects on society are among the least well known.

THE PREVALENCE OF CHRONIC PAIN IN CANADA ACCORDING TO AGE AND SEX

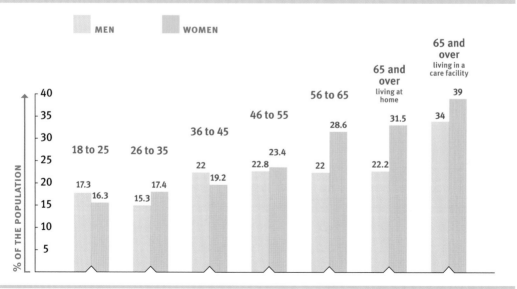

FIGURE 3   Schopflocher et al., 2011 ; Statistics Canada, 2008

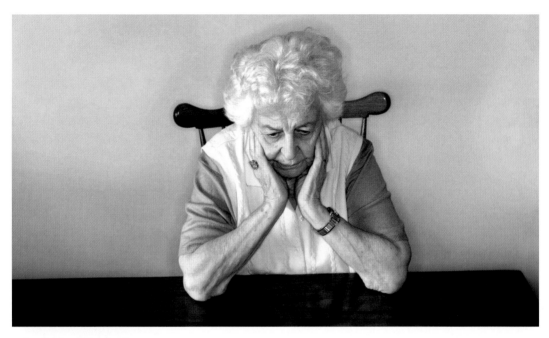

Is Pain Sexist?

Men and women experience pain differently. As a general rule, women report pain-related symptoms more often than men do. The pain tolerance threshold also seems to be lower in women than in men, particularly in terms of differences in temperature. This greater sensitivity could be related to the fact that in women the cutaneous nerve fibres are almost twice as dense as in men, which magnifies the intensity of the pain signal. Response to analgesic treatment also differs according to sex, with women having a therapeutic response noticeably greater than that of men, to opioids, for example. The causes of these differences are not yet fully understood, but they may indicate that sex hormones act differently on the mechanisms that integrate nociceptive stimuli in the brain: studies do in fact show that testosterone tends to decrease the perception of pain, while estrogen and progesterone, on the other hand, increase it (Gaumont and Marchand, 2006).

It must be remembered, however, that in addition to these physiological differences a number of sociocultural factors also contribute to the way in which pain is perceived by both sexes. Women in general pay more attention to their health, consult their doctor more regularly, and are often more comfortable discussing their experiences with respect to pain. While pain seems to be more common in women than in men, it remains a personal experience that varies a great deal more among individuals than according to their sex.

While chronic pain may seem to be a mysterious illness, its social repercussions could not be more concrete and measurable: in Canada alone, it's estimated that chronic pain costs approximately sixty billion dollars a year, an astronomical amount reflecting the heavy demand for health care from people who are ill, absenteeism at work, and the amounts spent on disability costs (Figure 4).

But aside from the direct economic costs it entails, chronic pain imposes physical, psychological and social pressures that can devastate the lives of sufferers and those of their family members. Pain is associated with a poor quality of life; its constant presence can totally disrupt every aspect of daily life — mood, sleep, nutrition — and lead to major changes, psychologically and in social relationships. It can even cause a deterioration in personality — including psychological problems and drug dependence. Clearly, chronic pain is a personal and social burden of unsuspected magnitude that we must understand more fully if we are to help sufferers feel better.

THE ROOTS OF PAIN

Before we can tackle the problem of chronic pain, we have to distinguish the various types of pain. Each type of pain is unique, strongly influenced by a wide range of physical, genetic, neurophysiological, environmental, emotional, and cultural factors specific to each of us. Nonetheless, the types of chronic pain can be grouped into four major categories, each with its own characteristics that will play a determining role in its treatment (Figure 5).

NOCICEPTIVE PAIN

This is caused by the overstimulation of pain receptors, called nociceptors. Chronic somatic pain involves the skin, muscles, and skeleton (bones, joints, tendons); chronic visceral pain affects the internal organs. Although this kind of pain is caused by excessive nociception, or too much stimulation of the sensory nerves, it manifests itself completely differently depending on the area of the body where the pain stimulus occurs. For example, somatic nociceptive pain is usually well localized and can be triggered by a movement or simply by touching, the best examples being osteoarthritis (degenerative arthritis) and rheumatoid arthritis. Visceral nociceptive pain, on the other hand, is harder to localize accurately and often takes the form of cramps or sudden stabbing pain that seems to go right through you.

THE ECONOMIC IMPACTS OF CHRONIC PAIN

Increased use of health care

4 medical visits/year for pain

Absenteeism at work

3.5 workdays/year (6 workdays in cases of severe pain)

Average median costs of care per person (before treatment in a pain clinic)

$1,462/month

Average global costs of care per person

$14,744/year

FIGURE 4   The Canadian Pain Society, 2011; Cherrière et al., 2010; Boulanger et al., 2007

Neuropathic Pain

Extremely complex and hard to treat, this kind of pain is caused by an attack on the nervous system — on the peripheral nerves, the spinal cord, or even the brain. This pain is usually described as a burning or tingling sensation that can reach peaks of intensity similar to those produced by an electrical discharge. Neuropathy resulting from diabetes or surgery is among the most frequent kinds of neuropathic pain.

MIXED PAIN

This pain is caused by the combined action of the factors responsible for nociceptive and neuropathic pain. Excessive nociception and an attack on the nervous system occurring at the same time cause very disabling chronic pain, leading to a major deterioration in quality of life. While mixed pain is common in patients with cancer, fibromyalgia and some types of lower back pain are the kinds of mixed pain that affect the largest number of people.

PSYCHOGENIC PAIN

Psychogenic pain is triggered by psychological factors and has no physical cause. This type of pain is quite rare in the general population and is not managed in the same way as neuropathic or nociceptive pain. It may occur in people with severe depression or in those with an emotional disorder manifesting itself physically as pain. Psychogenic pain is genuine pain in either a part of the body or the body as a whole. It's important, however, not to confuse psychogenic pain with the psychological aspects of chronic pain, such as those discussed later in this book.

THE MAIN TYPES OF CHRONIC PAIN

The types of chronic pain in each of these categories are found, to varying degrees, in the populations of industrialized countries. In Canada, back pain and joint diseases (osteoarthritis, arthritis) are the most common. Migraines are also a major source of chronic pain, and their prevalence is especially high in women (Figure 6). But these common ailments are not the only causes of chronic pain; for example, a recent enquiry among inhabitants of the European Union (*Pain Proposal*, 2010) shows that a significant portion of the European population has to deal with several distinct types of chronic pain, notably fibromyalgia, postoperative pain, and pain associated with diseases like diabetes or cancer (Figure 7). The high incidence and wide variety of chronic pain in the population eloquently illustrate the enormous challenge these diseases pose to our society.

BACK PAIN

Dubbed "the disease of the century" by some, lower back pain, or lumbago, strikes over 80 percent of the population sooner or later and is the main reason for visiting the doctor. In the vast majority of cases (90 percent), this back pain is a type of lumbago — the so-called "crick in the back" — a very painful ailment but one that usually disappears by itself in a few weeks. That said, 5 to 8 percent of cases of back pain become chronic and are accompanied by very disabling pain requiring significant changes in lifestyle for the sufferer, with all the socioeconomic repercussions

DIFFERENT TYPES OF PAIN

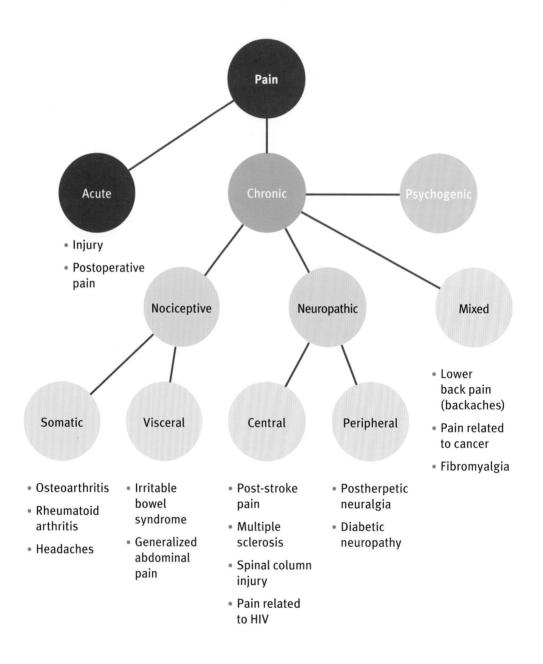

FIGURE 5

Schopflocher et al., 2011; Statistics Canada, 2008

that are unavoidably associated with such changes (Nguyen et al., 2009).

The high incidence of lower back pain shows just how vulnerable the part of the spinal column in the lower back is. The spinal column developed very early in the evolution of life; it consists of a series of vertebrae that, in all animal species, connect the front and back legs, creating a horizontal "bridge," whose main function is to support the weight of the internal organs. In human beings, however, the standing position completely changes the column's supporting role, as the vertebrae are stacked on top of each other and must therefore bear a considerable load. Since each vertebra bears the weight of the part of the body above it, the load is especially heavy for the five lumbar vertebrae, which must not only support the upper portions of the body (the head, shoulders, arms, and rib cage) and all the abdominal organs (stomach, intestines), but also whatever else a person is carrying. Not to mention

the foetus and eventually the baby in the case of a pregnant woman! Since the load on the lumbar region can feel like several hundred kilos when something heavy is being transported, this is an extremely fragile part of the body, mechanically speaking. This makes it more likely to suffer painful injuries.

The spinal column consists of seven cervical vertebrae in the neck, twelve dorsal vertebrae in the upper and middle parts of the trunk, and five lumbar vertebrae in its lower portion (Figure 8).

The column of vertebrae and discs is surrounded by a complex network of muscles, tendons and ligaments ensuring the stability and mobility of the spinal joints. Changes in any of these structures can cause back pain. For example, the stretching or tearing of ligaments next to the discs can cause a very painful sprain. However, it's the intervertebral discs that are especially vulnerable and a frequent cause of several kinds of back pain.

THE PREVALENCE OF CERTAIN CONDITIONS IN PEOPLE WITH CHRONIC PAIN, BY SEX, IN CANADA

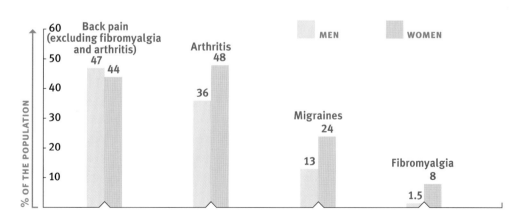

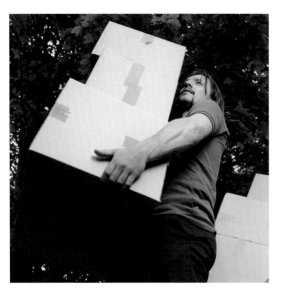

THE MAIN CAUSES OF CHRONIC PAIN: A EUROPEAN STUDY

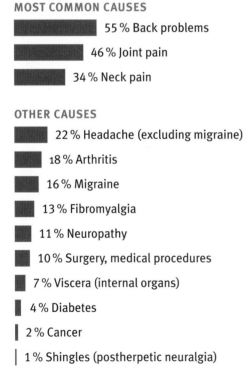

MOST COMMON CAUSES

55 % Back problems

46 % Joint pain

34 % Neck pain

OTHER CAUSES

22 % Headache (excluding migraine)

18 % Arthritis

16 % Migraine

13 % Fibromyalgia

11 % Neuropathy

10 % Surgery, medical procedures

7 % Viscera (internal organs)

4 % Diabetes

2 % Cancer

1 % Shingles (postherpetic neuralgia)

FIGURE 7   Pain Proposal — Improving the Current and Future Management of Chronic Pain, 2010

In people who put too heavy a load on their backs, notably by staying in the same position for a long time and performing movements that put too much strain on the vertebrae, the discs can deteriorate over time, lose their elastic properties, and become incapable of sufficiently absorbing shocks. In these circumstances, the vertebrae may begin to move around more than they should, requiring better muscle support to hold them in place, a form of compensation that often causes muscle spasms that "lock up" the back.

If a disc is damaged by an injury (a sudden movement, a load that's too heavy) or wear and tear, the jelly-like substance in the centre of the disc may bulge out of its normal space, pushing through the external layer and forming what's called a herniated disc or, in everyday language, "a slipped disc" (Figure 8). The hernia leads to the compression or inflammation of a nerve root (connected to the spinal cord running the entire length of the spinal column), thus causing very severe pain and a tearing sensation.

JOINT PAIN

A large proportion of patients with chronic pain have joint problems. In physiological terms, the movable joints, called synovial joints, are where two bones meet. They are constructed in such a way as to allow movements, while ensuring that adequate mechanical support is provided by ligaments. As a result, we place extremely heavy demands on these structures over a lifetime. To prevent premature wear and tear where the ends of the bones come into contact, they are covered by a layer of cartilage and surrounded by a viscous substance that looks like egg-white, called synovia; this "lubricates" the joint and ensures that it moves freely. While they are indispensable if our skeleton is to function smoothly, the joints are nonetheless fragile structures, susceptible to a wide range of problems caused by the inflammation of their constituent parts or by wear and tear.

What we call arthritis is in fact a generic term covering more than one hundred distinct diseases; all of them, however, share the common characteristic of causing pain in the musculoskeletal system, especially the joints, ligaments, and bones. The most common kinds of pain are those caused by osteoarthritis and rheumatoid arthritis, a disease that affects 4.2 million Canadians (16 percent of the population) aged fifteen and over. Given Canada's aging population, it's expected that this number will reach approximately seven million people (20 percent) by 2031 (Public Health Agency of Canada, 2010).

OSTEOARTHRITIS

Osteoarthritis, the most common type of arthritis, is characterized by a progressive deterioration of the joint cartilage that protects the bone, leaving it open to structural damage (Figure 9). This bone damage is often accompanied by the growth of bony projections called osteophytes on the edges of the joints, visible as lumps; it can be very painful and disabling, making it difficult to perform joint movements as basic as moving the fingers, turning the wrists or bending the knees. The pain associated with these movements can, indirectly, cause a decrease in mobility, leading to muscle atrophy and a

Michael, 32

Michael was a loader for over fifteen years. His job was to carry boxes of merchandise to the trucks that would take them across the country. One afternoon, when his workday was almost over, Michael heard a strange "crack" in his back while he was lifting a box, but he was nonetheless able to finish his workday without too much difficulty. Next morning, however, he felt a stabbing pain in his back and one leg that kept him from going to work. Medical examinations showed he had two herniated lumbar discs, as well as sciatic nerve compression. After six months of treatments, including anti-inflammatories and analgesics, his condition was not getting any better and Michael was still unable to return to work. There was even talk of surgery. Michael had to stop taking part in a number of sports and leisure activities he enjoyed. And he has had back pain ever since.

slackening of the ligaments, making the joint even weaker.

RHEUMATOID ARTHRITIS

In contrast to osteoarthritis, a joint disease caused by wear, rheumatoid arthritis is an auto-immune disorder resulting from an unwanted attack by the immune system on the synovial membranes covering the joints. When the inflammation of these membranes becomes chronic, cartilage and bone stiffen up and are gradually destroyed; this can cause intense pain and deform the joint.

THE SPINAL COLUMN

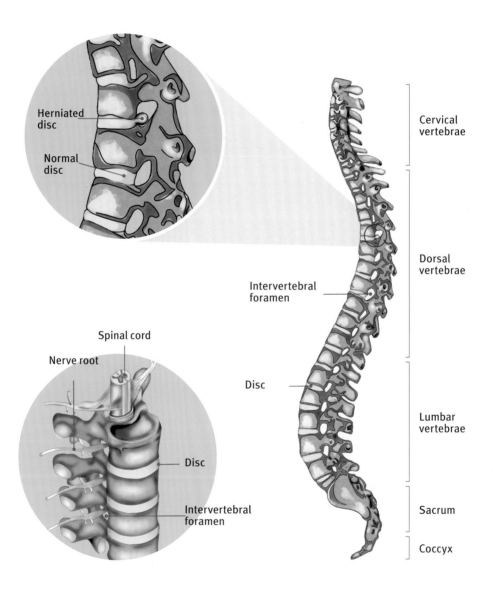

Herniated disc

Normal disc

Cervical vertebrae

Dorsal vertebrae

Intervertebral foramen

Spinal cord

Nerve root

Disc

Disc

Intervertebral foramen

Lumbar vertebrae

Sacrum

Coccyx

FIGURE 8

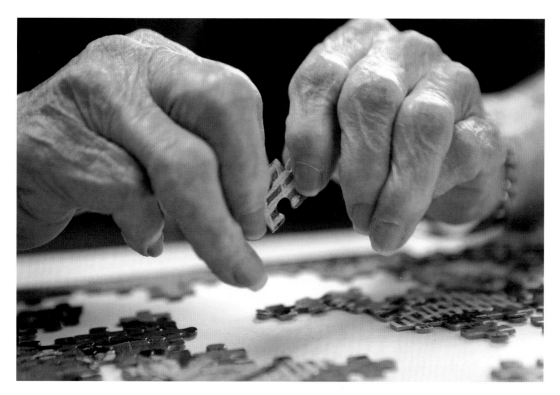

Even though we still know very little about the factors that trigger arthritis, it's thought that less than half of all cases are caused by genetic factors. Like several other chronic diseases (type 2 diabetes, cardiovascular disease), the development of arthritis may be related to certain lifestyle choices. For example, the increased pressure placed on the joints by excess weight seems to increase the risk of rheumatoid arthritis significantly, possibly because it involves premature wear and tear and the risk of inflammation.

NEUROPATHIC PAIN

The pain felt by people with neuropathic pain is typically burning or piercing, with violent and very incapacitating extremes. This kind of pain is usually associated

Teresa, 64

Teresa was a pastry chef and caterer for more than forty years. She devoted her life to serving her clients, but she has had to resign herself to slowing down her activities because of osteoarthritis in her hands, which is tormenting her more and more and from which she has suffered for nearly twenty years. She simply can no longer knead dough, roll it out and perform the movements needed to make the "little masterpieces" she was so proud of. She now realizes, to her great regret, that she will have to stop working. Her fingers were her whole life; from now on she will have to learn to live a new life without using her fingers the way she once did and to mourn the loss of what had always been the focal point of her life.

with a hypersensitivity to non-painful stimuli (for example, wearing clothes), a phenomenon known as allodynia, as well as a heightened response to stimuli that normally cause very little pain (hyperalgesia). This exhausting pain causes serious deterioration in quality of life for those afflicted.

In contrast to other types of pain triggered by injuries to a particular part of the body and transmitted to the brain by the nervous system (nociceptive pain), neuropathic pain is, by definition, caused by an injury to the nervous system itself, whether to the peripheral nerves, the spinal cord, or the brain. These nerve injuries may be caused by physical trauma (surgery, stroke, cancer), certain auto-immune diseases (multiple sclerosis), and metabolic disorders (diabetic neuropathies), or by infections (shingles). This range of factors makes neuropathic pain unique, both in terms of the intensity of the pain signal it sends and the wide array of body parts that may be affected.

Neuropathic pain brings into play complex physiopathological mechanisms, all of which have the ability to impair the functioning of nerve cells (neurons) significantly. However, injuries to nerves can't explain why, in some cases, pain persists in a particular area of the body long after an injury has healed, almost as if the body has stored the initial pain in its memory and continues to feel it with the same intensity as at the beginning.

Phantom limb pain is the best example of this phenomenon. Intuitively, it's perfectly logical to think that the amputation of a limb should eliminate the sensations that are normally felt in that part of the body. But such is not the case. The vast majority of amputees retain the memory of their limb in their "sensory memory" and feel like it's still there. Unfortunately, a high proportion of them also feel pain in this phantom limb — pain that may or may not be related to what caused the amputation.

OSTEOARTHRITIS

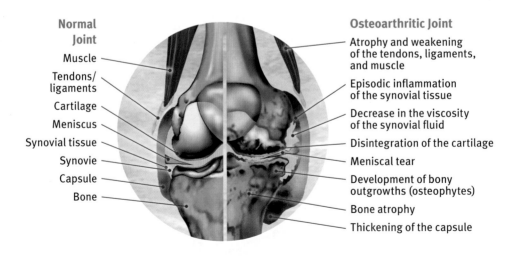

Normal Joint

Muscle
Tendons/ligaments
Cartilage
Meniscus
Synovial tissue
Synovie
Capsule
Bone

Osteoarthritic Joint

Atrophy and weakening of the tendons, ligaments, and muscle
Episodic inflammation of the synovial tissue
Decrease in the viscosity of the synovial fluid
Disintegration of the cartilage
Meniscal tear
Development of bony outgrowths (osteophytes)
Bone atrophy
Thickening of the capsule

FIGURE 9

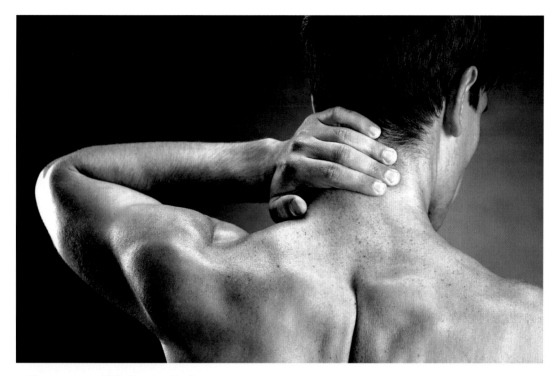

Hypersensitivity to Pain

Since the main function of pain is to protect the body from danger, one of the fundamental characteristics of injuries is that they remain sensitive for a while after healing in order to signal to the brain that it has to pay special attention to that particular part of the body. Sunburn doesn't threaten the health of a careless vacationer with immediate danger, but the nociceptors on the skin's sunburnt surface will certainly let the brain know that the area has been attacked and deserves special attention. This heightened sensitivity explains why the mere touch of fabric on the skin is felt with disproportionate intensity.

Allodynia is an extreme case where a sensation not normally thought to cause pain becomes painful. For example, for some people drafts from a fan feel like razor blades slashing their skin, or they suffer dreadfully if their skin comes into contact with just a lightweight piece of cloth. This mysterious phenomenon seems to be caused by a "reprogramming" of the nerves involved in transmitting the pain signal; harmless mechanical stimulation (like the contact of a piece of clothing with the skin) is treated as if it were dangerous, thus causing intense pain.

Hyperalgesia, on the other hand, is characterized by abnormally severe pain in response to a pain stimulus. In contrast to allodynia, hyperalgesia is caused by a magnification of the normal signal from pain receptors.

The perception of pain in the total absence of painful stimuli is caused by a "remapping" of the central nervous system in response to a peripheral injury. In fact, neurons are constantly rearranging themselves and never, throughout our entire lives, stop adapting to new demands. The malleability of neurons, called neuronal plasticity, makes it possible, for example, to learn a new language, or enables a musician or an athlete to create and maintain the neural circuits needed to master difficult routines. It's also because of neuronal plasticity that victims of brain trauma, a stroke for example, can learn to speak and move all over again, as the neurons in the healthy regions of the brain take on new responsibilities to compensate for the loss of function in damaged cells. Phantom limb pain shows, however, that this neuronal plasticity is not always helpful, since the damage to the peripheral nerve fibres caused by amputation triggers, in several areas of the nervous system, a neuronal reorganization that disrupts the way the brain perceives the body (Elbert, 2011).

More than any other kind of pain, neuropathic pain is thus the tangible expression of the complex mechanisms at play in transmitting the pain signal and the brain's central role in perceiving this pain.

HEADACHES

The most common chronic headaches are tension headaches, so called because they result from stress or muscular and skeletal problems in the neck area. The pain is constant and it feels like the head is being squeezed in a vise; it can sometimes last several days. While the mechanisms underlying these headaches are still poorly understood, a number of triggering factors have been identified

Migraines are the other most common type of chronic headache, affecting 15 percent of women and 7 percent of men in Canada (Statistics Canada, 2007–2008). They typically cause intense pain, usually on only one side of the head (the word migraine comes from the Greek *êmikranion*, meaning "pain on one side of the head") and are usually accompanied by nausea or vomiting, as well as a hypersensitivity to light and noise. In roughly a third of sufferers, the migraine is preceded by sensory disturbances called "auras," the most common being phosphenes (flashes), scotomas (blotchy vision), or various geometric shapes and flashes.

Although they don't pose any immediate danger to health, migraines are very painful and hard to treat, and prevention remains therefore by far the best weapon at the disposal of people who get them. Most migraine sufferers learn to identify one or

Peter, 56

Peter's life was turned upside down by a serious stroke (also called a cerebrovascular accident or CVA). Since then, he has had episodes of extremely intense pain in the entire left side of his body, like a burning sensation or electrical shocks in the arm and numbness in the leg and foot. The pain in his arm is such that he has to wear a splint all the time to keep it from touching his clothing, as well as to let people he meets know that they are not to touch his arm.

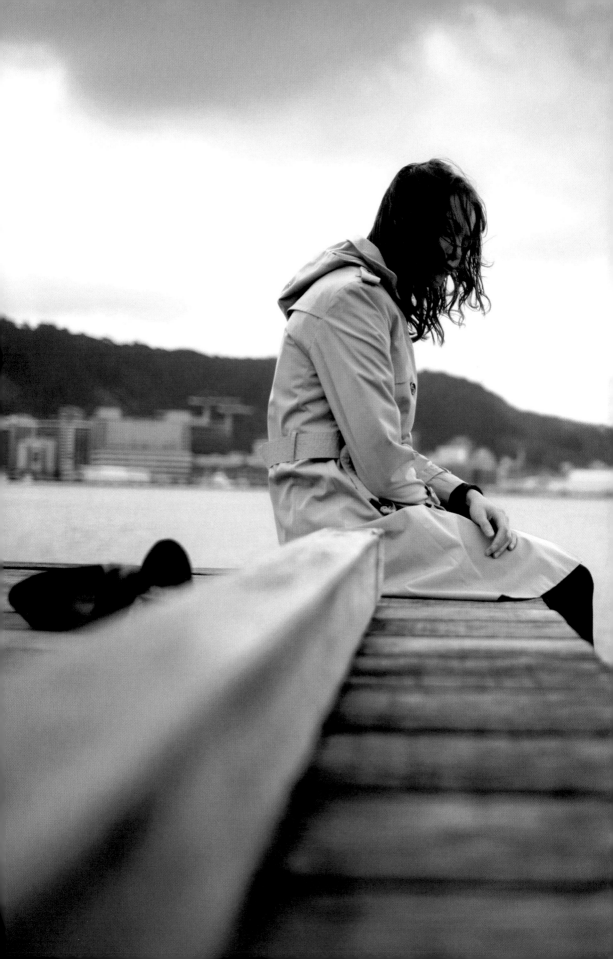

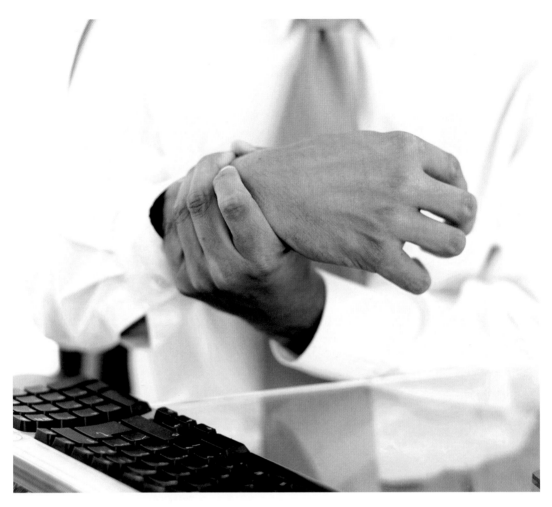

Frayed Nerves

Since nerves are the cornerstone of the pain transmission system, it goes without saying that attacks on these structures can cause many different kinds of pain. In addition to the most common attacks on the nervous system, in particular post-operative trauma, a certain number of less common illnesses can cause extremely intense pain that turns sufferers' everyday lives upside down.

Burning Mouth Syndrome
Stomatodynia, better known as "burning mouth syndrome," is a type of chronic pain characterized by spontaneous and continuous burning sensations in the mucous membranes of the mouth despite there being no obvious injury. This type of neuropathic pain is particularly common in women (seven women for every man), with 90 percent of patients being menopausal. The causes remain

vague but appear to involve a malfunction in the nerves transmitting trigeminal sensory information (temperature, texture, astringency) and the sensation of taste (Minor and Epstein, 2011).

Carpal Tunnel Syndrome

A very common neuropathy found in millions of people around the world, this syndrome is caused by compression of the median nerve in the wrist. This nerve, connecting the hand to the forearm, runs through the carpal tunnel, a triangular space surrounded by bone and conjunctive tissue.

A number of lifestyle-related factors, especially performing repetitive manual activities and being overweight, can cause the tunnel to narrow, compressing the nerve and impeding the flow of the nerve impulse. This compression is felt as numbness or tingling (Luckhaupt et al., 2010).

Postherpetic Neuralgia (Shingles)

Chicken pox is a common and highly contagious childhood disease caused by the varicella zoster virus (VZV), a close cousin of the virus that causes herpes. After infection, the virus settles into the sensory nerve ganglions, where it can lie dormant for decades before becoming active again and causing a localized skin eruption (shingles). When it's reactivated in the ganglions, the virus destroys the nerves in the area, resulting in itching and severe pain that can last for a long time — sometimes more than six months — after the dermatosis has disappeared (Schmader, 2002).

Diabetic Neuropathy

Diabetes is a state of chronic hyperglycemia occurring when the pancreas is unable to produce insulin or the organs are unable to absorb sugar in response to insulin.

High blood sugar levels damage the cells of the organism in many ways and can in the long-term change the way nerve cells function. Approximately 50 percent of diabetics experience these attacks on the nerve fibres. They cause very sharp pain in the arms, legs, hands and feet, as well as allodynia, an extreme sensitivity to even the most harmless contact (Schmader, 2002).

Cancer

Half of cancer patients live with moderate to severe pain, which becomes much worse in the most advanced stages of the disease.

In addition to pain caused by pressure on the nerves from the mass of cancer cells, the rapid progression of tumours and the various destructive enzymes they secrete frequently result in nerve damage and pain pathway activation (see Chapter 2) (Portenoy, 2011).

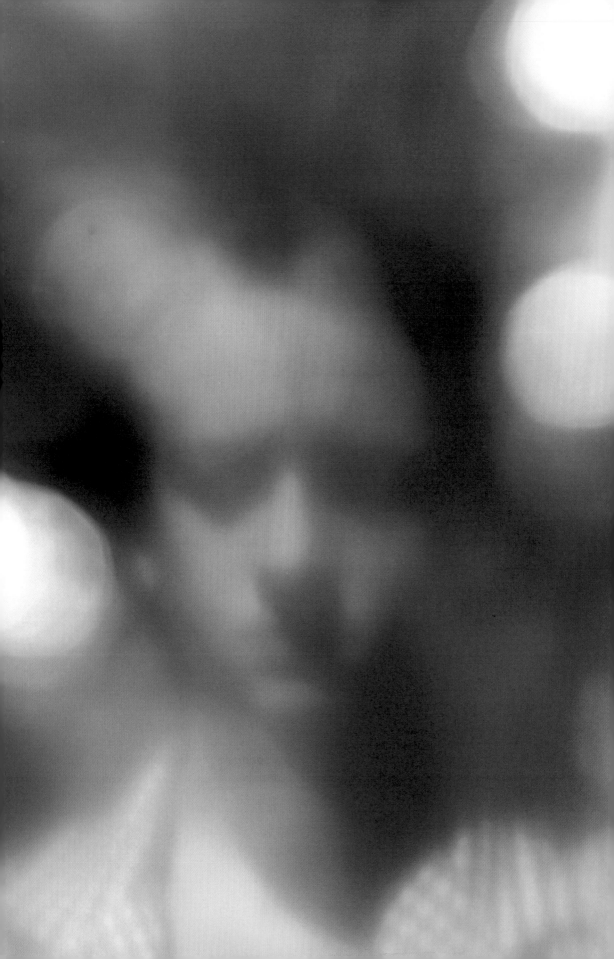

more risk factors that increase their risk of getting a migraine (Figure 10), and making changes in lifestyle to avoid being exposed to these factors often makes a reduction in the frequency and (or) intensity of the attacks possible.

VISCERAL PAIN

Sooner or later everyone gets a stomach ache, which usually doesn't last very long and has no negative impact on health. Women are particularly familiar with "normal" visceral pain, since the major physiological changes that are part of their reproductive cycle (menstrual cycle, childbirth, menopause) are often associated with episodes of pain.

Sometimes, however, abdominal pain becomes more severe, causing cramps or pain in a large portion of the abdomen or in the pelvic area. Painful periods (dysmenorrhea), genital and urinary infections, and irritable bowel syndrome are jointly responsible for a large proportion of this visceral pain, but acute pain caused by potentially deadly illnesses like heart attack (myocardial infarction), acute pancreatitis, and peritonitis is also significant.

The location and intensity of visceral pain varies considerably depending on the affected organ, making accurate diagnosis difficult. These unique characteristics stem from major differences in the nerve fibre circuits connecting the internal organs to the brain. For example, the stomach, intestines, bladder and uterus contain a great many sensory nerve fibres; this means that an attack — even a minor one — on these organs can trigger great pain. In contrast, other organs like the liver, kidneys, and

THE MAIN TRIGGERERING FACTORS FOR HEADACHES

Tension Headaches
- Over-consumption of medication
- Poor posture at work or during sleep, especially if this affects the neck and shoulder muscles
- Fatigue caused by lack of sleep or too much work
- Eating very cold food (ice cream, for example)
- Dental problems (clicking jaws, grinding teeth) caused by a malfunctioning temporomandibular joint (this is known as temporomandibular joint disorder, a complaint that can be related to many forms of head and facial pain)

Migraines
- Stress and anxiety
- Changes of season
- Caffeine (more or less than usual), chocolate, alcohol (often red wine)
- Lack of or too much sleep, fatigue
- Hormonal changes related to the menstrual cycle
- Skipping a meal
- Certain foods containing nitrates (cold meats, for example), tyramine (aged cheeses, smoked fish), monosodium glutamate, or aspartame

FIGURE 10   Adapted from Hildreth, Lynm, Glass, 2009

Amber, 54

For twenty-five years, Amber has suffered from recurring headaches that occur mainly in stressful situations. The pain feels like a sort of band around her head, particularly on the left side around the eye and the arch of the eyebrow. When this happens, she has to take very powerful painkillers to ease the pain. During these attacks, Amber can't get out of bed and has to stay away from work and cancel her activities. Although over the years she has managed to identify certain factors that trigger her headaches, Amber lives in constant fear of an unexpected attack.

Joyce, 44

Joyce has suffered from abdominal pain for fifteen years. She has cramps as well as constant pain in the abdomen. She has frequent spells of constipation, alternating with diarrhea. This situation makes her very ill at ease in public, since she can't predict how she will feel. Joyce manages to decrease or avoid some kinds of pain by watching her diet. However, she is always in some pain and this keeps her from functioning normally. She frequently has to stay home from work and has stopped participating in a number of physical activities, as she feels tired and has no energy.

lungs contain very few nociceptive fibres. This is why some serious illnesses involving these organs can remain asymptomatic until their functioning deteriorates to the point of jeopardizing the person's overall state of health.

FIBROMYALGIA

Fibromyalgia is a syndrome consisting of generalized aches and pains throughout the body, usually accompanied by tremendous fatigue and sleep disturbances, as well as episodes of anxiety or depression. This is a very difficult illness to diagnose, since several of its symptoms resemble those of other illnesses, in particular chronic fatigue syndrome and irritable bowel syndrome. Until fairly recently, the main diagnostic technique was to palpate eighteen tender points all over the body to determine the resulting level of pain; the sensation of pain at eleven or more points was considered to be a sign of fibromyalgia. Since 2010, however, these tender points have no longer been used, as studies have shown that people with fibromyalgia have heightened sensitivity in all areas of the body (Wolfe et al., 2010). Diagnosis now takes greater account of other symptoms of the disease, such as fatigue, disrupted sleep, and various cognitive impacts.

Widespread pain throughout the body, as well as hypersensitivity to most stimuli (warmth, cold, electric shock, light, noise), suggests that fibromyalgia is a disorder caused by an attack on the nervous system that magnifies pain perception.

We still know very little about the factors that cause fibromyalgia. We do know, however, that there is a strong family

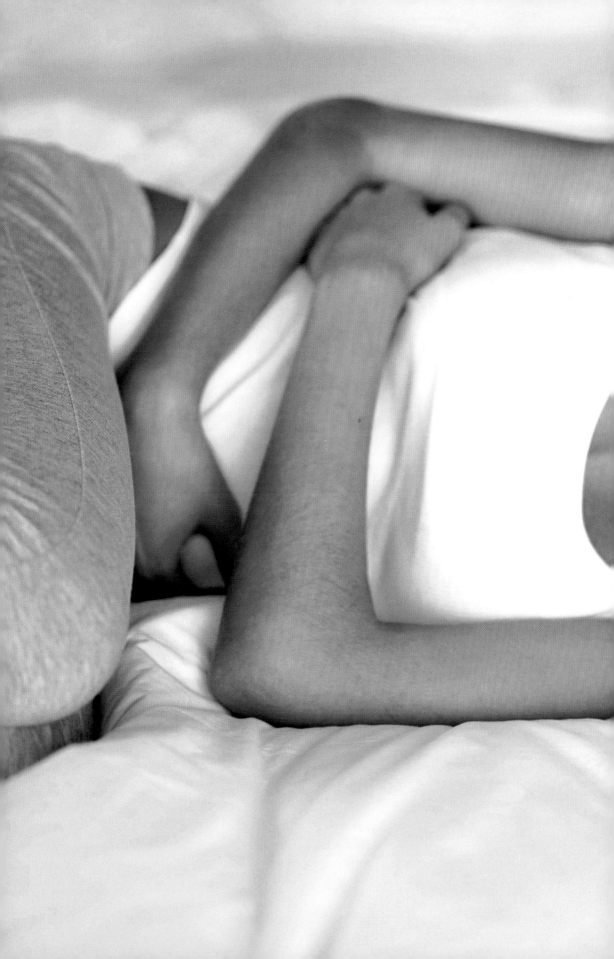

Chloe, 38

Eight years ago, Chloe was in a car accident and suffered various injuries that she has partially recovered from. At the time of the accident, she experienced great stress and feared for her life. Since then, Chloe has had pain all over her body that sometimes moves from one area to another. On some days, her body is so stiff she can hardly move. She feels constantly exhausted, can no longer get a satisfying night's sleep and feels more and more depressed. Chloe feels she's a prisoner in a body that's becoming less and less able to do things.

predisposition, the risk being eight times higher for people who have a close relative with the disease (parents, brothers, or sisters). As is the case for other kinds of pain, women seem more susceptible to it than men, with a risk four times higher. Stress, both psychological and physiological, also plays a role in the development of the disease. A high level of psychological stress, combined with overwhelming events such as the tragic death of a loved one or serious trauma, increases the risk of suffering from fibromyalgia (Staud et al., 2009).

This overview has outlined the many different kinds of chronic pain, as well as the considerable impact it has on the well-being of the population. Pain is still a mysterious experience that presents a serious challenge to human understanding. Why do we become ill? Why do medical treatments not succeed in relieving our ailments?

To answer these questions, we need to know more about the mechanisms underlying the pain sensation; we have to understand just how complex the pain phenomenon is, especially when it becomes chronic, and how many physiological and psychological processes are involved. While pain is first and foremost a physical sensation, the fact remains that its perception — in other words, the way people experience it — is dramatically influenced by various sociocultural factors specific to a given time period or culture. Welcome to the mysterious world of pain.

In Summary

- In Canada, one person in five has to deal with persistent pain on a daily basis, making chronic illness our society's most widespread disease.

- Chronic pain can occur throughout the entire body, although back pain, arthritis, and migraine are the most frequent types.

- This pain causes a major deterioration in the quality of life of sufferers.

- The high prevalence of chronic pain entails a very high socio-economic cost.

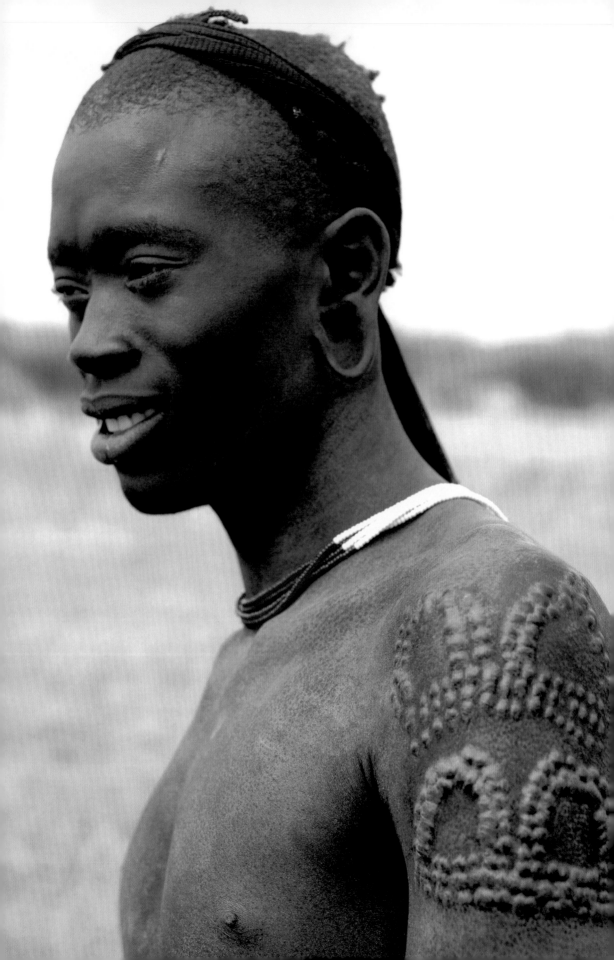

CHAPTER 2

Pain Under the Magnifying Glass

There is no more lively sensation than that of pain.
— MARQUIS DE SADE

We interact with our surroundings by means of very sophisticated detection systems that can decode information found in the environment and convert it into signals that are transmitted to certain very specific regions in the brain for interpretation. The primary function of the five senses — sight, taste, smell, hearing, and touch — is therefore mainly to keep the brain in constant contact with the outside world, so that it can quickly offer an "opinion" on how to behave in a positive or negative situation.

Detecting these sensations, however, is only the physical part of an infinitely more complex process. Being dazzled by the beauty of an artist's work or a magnificent landscape is not just about simply looking at these things; feeling intense emotion while listening to a melody played by a musician is not simply the result of listening to a sound, any more

than the pleasure associated with the delicious flavour of a dish stems from ingesting a particular food. It is instead a matter of interpreting these sensations, of perceiving them in a way that gives them a dimension extending far beyond a simple physical sense. If it weren't for perception, everything around us would be neither beautiful nor ugly, music would be just a nondescript mixture of sounds, and everything we eat would simply be a source of energy. In other words, while the basic function of the nervous system is to collect sensory information, the phenomenal development of the brain means we can add an emotional dimension that gives it meaning. These perceptions vary considerably according to each person's genetic and cultural baggage and reflect the very essence of our personality, the tangible expression of the evolution of our brain, and the sensitivity of our soul.

WHAT IS PAIN?

This distinction between sensation and perception is important in trying to understand pain. Although the sensation produced by a pain signal is nearly identical from one person to another, the *perception* of this sensation, or the way the sensation is interpreted by the brain, can vary depending on the individual, the time period, and the culture. The contribution of the physical senses and emotions to the phenomenon of pain is well illustrated in the definition proposed by the International Association for the Study of Pain: "[Pain is] an unpleasant sensory and emotional experience associated with actual or potential tissue damage, or described in terms of such damage."

This definition summarizes the vast range of sensations and emotions experienced by people who have to cope with pain. It's undeniable that pain is the result of some internal or external physical trauma producing intense pain signals that require urgent medical attention for relief. This is the sensory component of pain — what we call nociception. However, pain is not just an objective response to these sensations; as we have seen, it's common for people to live everyday with persistent pain, even when there's no damage or long after an injury has healed, just as others have injuries but no pain. It's clear that what we call "pain" is far more than nociception alone; it also has a powerful subjective and emotional component.

To understand pain fully, therefore, we have to examine not only the mechanisms that cause the pain sensation, but also look carefully at how emotions can change our

Sensation and Perception

Sensation is a raw physical phenomenon, received by the nervous system as important information to analyze but which hasn't yet been interpreted by the brain.

Perception is the brain's overall interpretation of a sensation, a phenomenon strongly influenced by sociocultural context and emotions.

Nociception and Pain

Nociception is the sensory process that generates the nerve message and causes pain.

Pain is the perception of this sensation, an interpretation by the brain influenced by several cognitive and emotional factors.

perception of this sensation and the intensity of the pain experienced.

AN ALARM SIGNAL

Like all physical sensations, the process of detecting and interpreting pain relies on several hundred billion nerve cells that interact with each other to form a high-performance communication network able to integrate and quickly handle a multitude of different pieces of information. The basic unit of the nervous system is the neuron, a kind of hyperspecialized cell that can generate, transmit, and receive information in the form of electrochemical signals. Nerve impulses coming from an injury site, whether internal or external, travel to the brain, alerting it to the fact that the body's well-being is under attack and telling it where on the body the trauma has occurred, so that it can order an appropriate response.

To visualize the importance of this alarm system, picture the head of a security squad whose job is to coordinate the movements of various guards in a huge building, while remaining confined in an isolated room. A task like this is impossible to carry out without communicating with the outside world; the leader has to use "sensors" (cameras, microphones, heat sensors) that pick up everything that's going on in the immediate environment and then give orders depending on the nature of the signals received. The system that responds to attacks on the smooth functioning of the organism is similar. Physically isolated from the rest of the body in the skull, the brain, the "head" that controls all of the physiological processes essential for life, has to rely on the nervous system, on its "sensors," which keep it informed in real time of events occurring in every part of the body so that it can react quickly to a potential threat.

To send a signal from the periphery to a particular region of the brain, the body has developed a very precise communication system based on close coordination between the two main parts of the nervous system, the central nervous system, and the peripheral nervous system, each specializing in a particular task (Figure 12).

The part of the peripheral nervous system involved in sensation is made up of a complex network of nerve fibres found throughout the organism. Its role is to collect information coming from both inside and outside the body. The central nervous system, meanwhile, consists of the brain, responsible for integrating and interpreting signals from the periphery, and the spinal cord. Actually an extension of the brain, the spinal cord acts as a relay station for transmitting signals from most of the peripheral nerves and in this way plays a key role in integrating the sensations that cause pain.

The way the nervous system is organized to detect and react to pain is absolutely remarkable in its efficiency. For example, if a sharp pebble gets into a walker's shoe, pressure and rubbing on the skin activate the nerves in the area; these then generate a nerve impulse that goes first to the spinal cord and from there to the regions of the brain specialized to handle this information — the somatosensory cortex, for one. Alerted to the threat, the brain then sends a nerve impulse via the spinal cord in the opposite direction. This reaches the muscles controlling the movements of the foot and stops it from landing too heavily on the ground, thus decreasing friction from the pebble, which would cause a limp. The entire process takes place in a fraction of a second, quickly putting an end to a situation that could lead to other injuries if it continued.

Pain can therefore be considered first of all as a very efficient alarm signal able to detect a peripheral threat and quickly alert the brain. Although pain is felt physically, it's also a "cerebral" phenomenon: it isn't the foot that feels pain because of the pebble, it's the brain! Indeed, if it weren't for the interpretation of the nerve impulse caused by the pebble's pressure, this threat wouldn't be noticed. The central nervous system's role is especially well illustrated

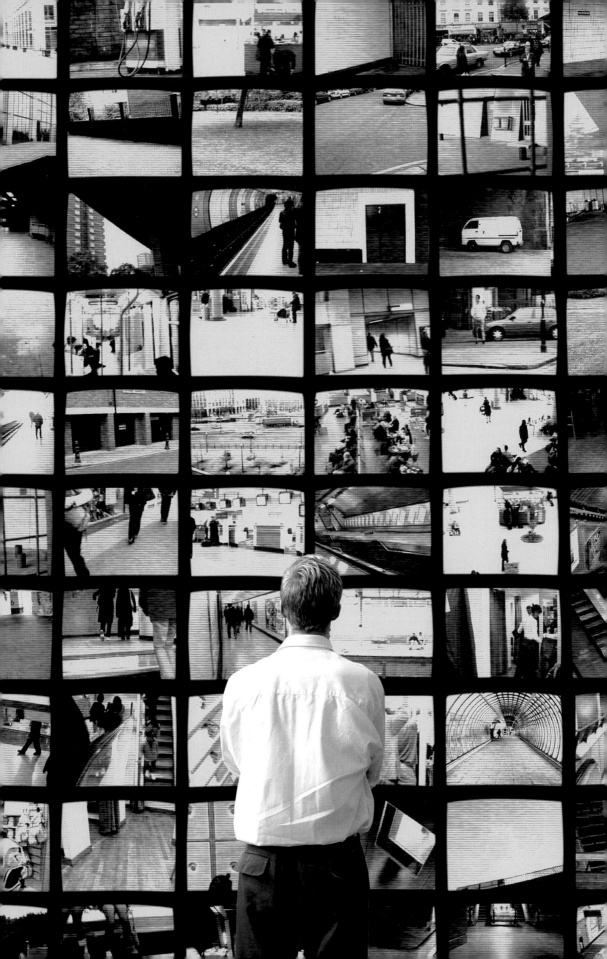

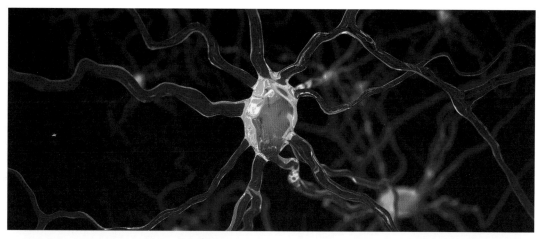

Putting Our Neurons to Work

Neurons are very special cells with two types of extensions, dendrites and axons, located at each end of the cell. This unique configuration makes the neurons the ultimate "social" cells, since they can interact with a multitude of other neurons through connections called synapses: a single neuron creates an average of ten thousand synapses by means of its dendrites and its axon! With its approximately 100 billion neurons, the human brain contains roughly a million billion (10^{15}) of these connections. This is truly a "social network" of unimaginable complexity; it works behind the scenes to coordinate every aspect of our existence — our movements, thoughts, and sensations.

In response to a given stimulus, neurons generate electrical activity and then transmit it as a nerve impulse to other neurons. The speed of this nerve impulse varies greatly depending on the diameter of the nerve fibres and whether they are myelinated. Myelin is a substance that acts as an insulating sheath and considerably speeds up nerve impulse transmission. In the case of signals related to pain, there are two distinct types of nerve fibres: A-delta fibres have a larger diameter and are covered in myelin; they transmit stabbing pain signals (an intense burn, for example) quickly. C fibres are smaller in diameter and lack myelin; they're responsible for the dull pain that follows the initial sharp pain and lasts long after the attack is over (Figure 11).

Nerve fibres and nerves must not be confused: a nerve fibre is the axon of a single neuron, whereas a nerve is a grouping of many of these nerve fibres (up to five hundred thousand), whose function is to bring together in the same structure a group of neurons linking the brain to a specific part of the human body. The nerves that transmit information from the periphery to the brain are called sensory (or afferent) nerves, while those that work in the opposite direction and carry the brain's orders to the periphery are called motor (or efferent) nerves. That said, most nerves are "mixed," that is, they contain both sensory and motor nerve fibres.

NERVE IMPULSE TRANSMISSION

A-delta fibres have a large diameter, transmit nerve impulses very quickly and are responsible for sharp and instant pain. C fibres have a smaller diameter and therefore transmit nerve impulses more slowly; they cause the dull pain that lingers after contact with the stimulus.

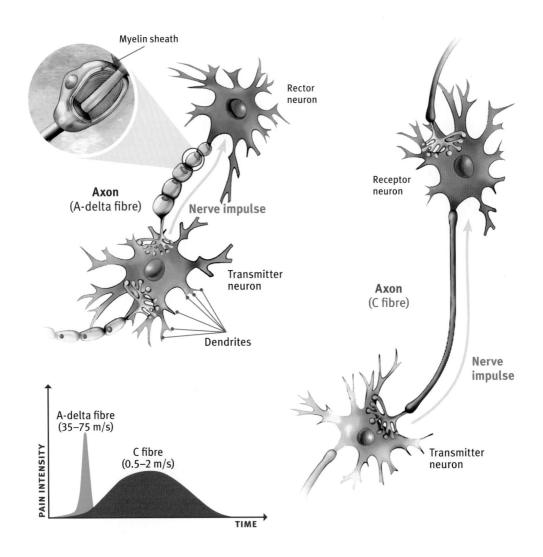

FIGURE 11

THE NERVOUS SYSTEM

The human nervous system is composed of the central nervous system (brain and spinal cord) and the peripheral nervous system (nerves). The nerves consist of several thousand neuronal extensions (axons) that transmit information.

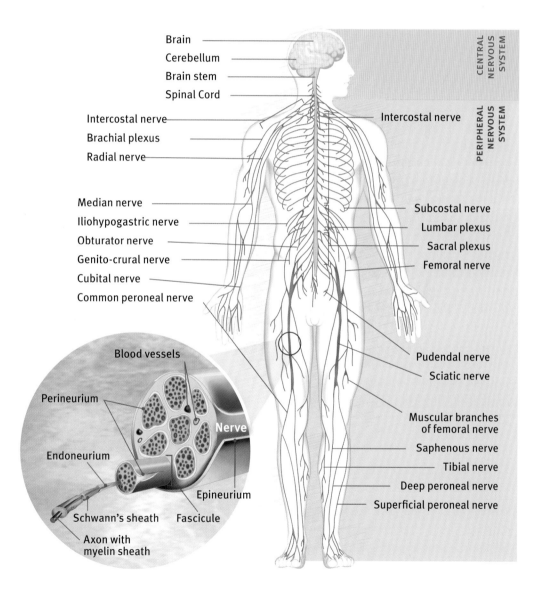

FIGURE 12

A Life Without Pain

In terms of pain sensation, congenital insensitivity to pain is one of the most curious neurological impairments. People with this very rare genetic disorder can perceive all physical sensations (touch, temperature, pressure), but are insensitive to painful stimuli. Without this protective signal, these people are at risk of injuries (bites, burns, fractures) that can cause disability, as well as serious or deadly infections.

Lack of sensitivity to pain doesn't just indicate poor functioning of the sensory nerves. People who have pain asymbolia, a condition usually caused by brain trauma, feel a pain stimulus physically, but are not bothered by it. The reasons for this indifference remain unclear, but recent studies indicate that it may be related to damage to the insular cortex and the anterior cingulate cortex, two regions of the brain that are partly responsible for awareness and the integration of emotions. The person therefore retains the ability to receive the pain message, but can no longer understand the signal indicating that the body's well-being is under threat.

in certain neurological disorders where people don't feel any pain following disruptions in the transmission or reception of a painful nerve impulse (see "A Life Without Pain," above). Just like all other physical sensations, what we call "pain" is in reality a perception, our brain's interpretation of a physical sensation signalling the presence of something dangerous.

ONWARD TO THE BRAIN!

The crucial role of the brain in pain perception requires secure lines of communication that can quickly and accurately transmit information from the periphery. To illustrate as concretely as possible the broad outlines of how these mechanisms work, let's take the pain from a burn as an example — pain we are only too familiar with. There are three main stages involved in the pain sensation: activation, transmission through the spinal cord, and arrival in the brain.

ACTIVATION

To be felt, pain must first be detected. This is the job of multiple nerve fibres located under the surface of the skin. On the ends of these fibres are nociceptors, a class of receptor proteins that can recognize a nociceptive stimulus (such as too much heat) and convert it into an electrical message relayed to the brain to inform it of the threat.

All of us who've burned ourselves know that the burning sensation occurs in two successive phases, with the initial sudden pain giving way within minutes to a duller and more generalized pain that can last several days. The immediate pain is caused by the activation of the fast-conducting fibres (A-delta), whose signal quickly alerts the brain as to the exact spot that has come into contact with the heat source. The dull pain that persists long after the heat source has been removed is transmitted by slower fibres (C fibres). This older detection system is responsible in particular for the emotional aspect of pain — the awareness that it's unpleasant and should be avoided as much as possible.

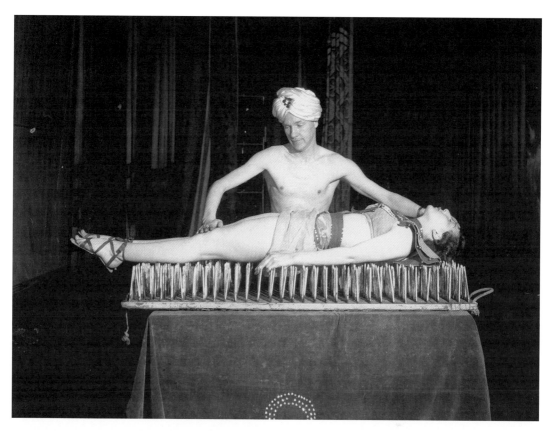

Nociceptors: The Pain Antennas

The human body has many nociceptors that act as antennas to detect harmful conditions, such as too much mechanical pressure, a temperature that's too high or too low, or chemical irritants released after trauma or produced by inflammation.

Some organs have more nociceptors than others and are therefore more sensitive to pain. The skin, which is in direct contact with the external environment and more susceptible to injury, is the organ in the body with the greatest number of these receptors, which are especially concentrated in the hands and feet. Other organs such as the testicles are highly innervated and also very sensitive, whereas the liver, spleen, and lungs are the source of very little pain. One curious thing is that the brain has no nociceptors whatsoever and therefore cannot feel pain. When we have a headache, it's not the brain that's affected, but rather the blood vessels in the head. Interestingly, this property can be put to good advantage in removing certain brain tumours: keeping patients awake during an operation makes constant monitoring of their cognitive functions possible (language, reading), so that contact with the regions of the brain performing these functions is avoided.

THE REFLEX ARC

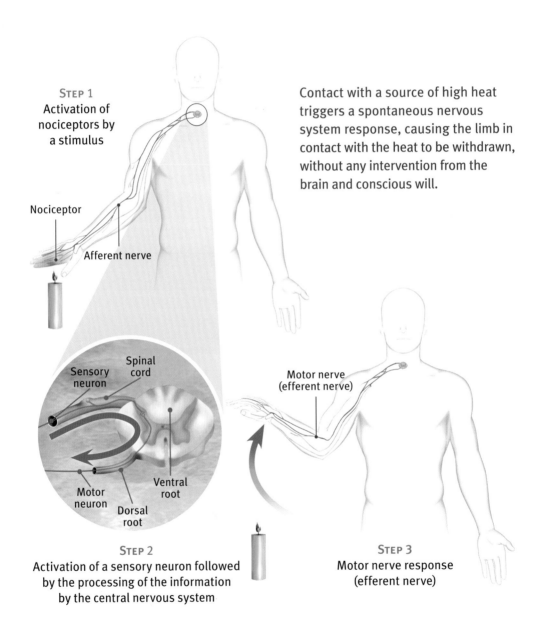

STEP 1
Activation of
nociceptors by
a stimulus

Contact with a source of high heat
triggers a spontaneous nervous
system response, causing the limb in
contact with the heat to be withdrawn,
without any intervention from the
brain and conscious will.

Nociceptor

Afferent nerve

Spinal
cord

Sensory
neuron

Motor nerve
(efferent nerve)

Motor
neuron

Ventral
root

Dorsal
root

STEP 2
Activation of a sensory neuron followed
by the processing of the information
by the central nervous system

STEP 3
Motor nerve response
(efferent nerve)

FIGURE 13

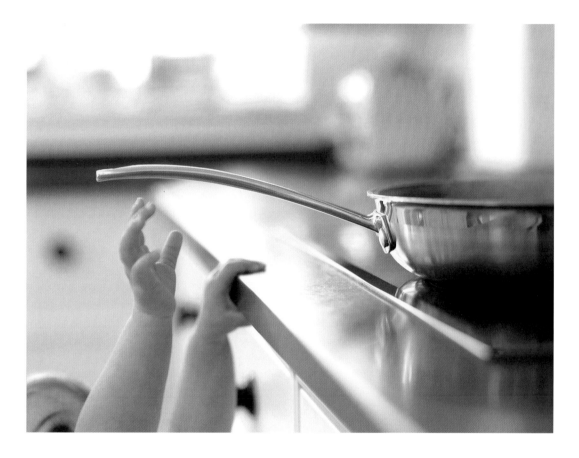

THE SPINAL CORD: A SORTING CENTRE

Tucked away in the centre of the spinal column, the spinal cord is the sorting centre for the nervous system, the place where signals from the peripheral nerves are received and carefully sorted before being transmitted to the brain.

What happens in the spinal cord is closely related to the kind of nerve impulses received. To continue with the preceding example, the impulses transmitted by fast and slow nerve fibres first enter the spinal cord via the dorsal root, a "gateway" in the rear part of the cord (on the side toward the back), and transmit the information to relay neurons in the area. If the signal these neurons receive exceeds a certain sensitivity threshold, in response to contact with a source of intense heat such as a red-hot stove burner, for example, the signal is immediately transmitted to a motor nerve so as to trigger an immediate muscular contraction and cause the hand to be withdrawn (Figure 13). This system, called the reflex arc, triggers a lightning-fast reaction to a dangerous situation in order to limit damage, even before the brain has understood that this is a pain signal. This is essential, for although nerve impulse transmission is fast, the time needed for the round trip to the brain and back still takes nearly a second, a delay in response that's too long and might result in significantly more damage to the body.

Contact with an intense heat source thus triggers a spontaneous response from the nervous system, causing the limb in contact with the heat to be immediately withdrawn, without the intervention of the brain or conscious will.

However, the nerve fibres activated by the heat do more than simply trigger the reflex arc. Their role is to alert the brain to the danger the body is facing, and they therefore have to spell each other off so the message can be delivered. The path taken by the impulse is convoluted (Figure 14): the signal transported by the two kinds of fibres (fast and slow) first changes direction and travels to the opposite side of the cord. This is a phenomenon, known as decussation, which causes the sensations received on the right side of the body to be handled by the left hemisphere of the central nervous system and vice versa.

Only once it reaches the opposite side of the spinal cord can the second neuron actually access the pathways that will allow it to travel all the way up the cord to the brain stem and the brain. These pathways differ, depending on the kind of nerve fibres transporting the signal: the fastest neurons (A-delta) use an "express" path that goes directly to the brain without stopping in other structures of the nervous system. This spinothalamic pathway appeared quite recently in evolutionary terms and serves mainly to carry information telling the brain about the source and intensity of the pain. The slower fibres (C fibres), on the other hand, use the older paleospinothalamic pathway and only reach the brain after passing through several regions of the brain stem, the structure located between the spinal cord and the brain.

REACHING THE BRAIN

The different pathways taken by fast and slow nerve impulses obviously have major repercussions on the kind of message carried to the brain. By taking the direct "express" pathway, the nerve impulse transmitted by fast fibres goes directly to the thalamus, the region of the brain essential for sorting and transmitting sensory information to the appropriate areas of the brain. When the message carried by the fast fibres reaches this structure, it's immediately deciphered and relayed to a third neuron connected to the primary somatosensory cortex (SI), a region that is like a topographical map of the body for locating bodily sensations. By stimulating this region of the brain, the fast A-delta fibres can therefore, in barely a few tenths of a second, send a strong pain signal in response to a harmful stimulus and indicate what kind of pain it is, thus allowing the brain to determine the exact location of the burn.

The slow fibres, which developed at a much earlier stage in the evolutionary process, don't use this tracking system; this is why the signal transmitted by these fibres is associated with more generalized "emotional" pain, whose primary aim is to communicate the unpleasant side of pain and the danger associated with it. Instead of reaching the thalamus directly via the "express" pathway, slow fibres use a secondary route that passes through the many structures in the brain stem. Just like when we travel on small country roads and ask regularly for directions, taking this secondary route is likely to lead to numerous encounters with certain neurons that modify, sometimes in surprising ways, the intensity of the response to a painful stimulus.

THE PAIN SIGNAL PATHWAYS

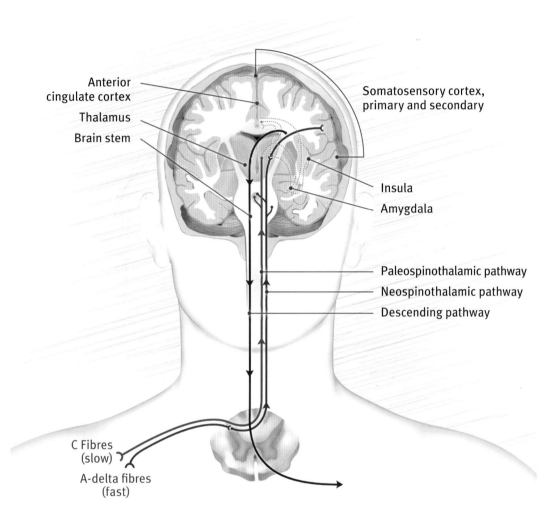

Anterior cingulate cortex
Thalamus
Brain stem

Somatosensory cortex, primary and secondary

Insula
Amygdala

Paleospinothalamic pathway
Neospinothalamic pathway
Descending pathway

C Fibres (slow)
A-delta fibres (fast)

The pain signal can reach the brain via two pathways, depending on the type of nerve fibre stimulated, A-delta or C. These are the ascending pain pathways: the neospinothalamic pathway and the paleospinothalamic pathway.

When it reaches the brain, the signal circulates to various regions as well as to the brain stem; these parts of the brain modulate the signal and control its intensity. This is the descending pathway.

FIGURE 14

Only after all the information from the brain stem has been assimilated will the signal transmitted by the slow fibres finally reach a distinct region of the thalamus. From there it will be relayed to several parts of the brain, including the secondary somatosensory cortex (SSC), insular cortex and the anterior cingulate cortex, the latter two regions being responsible for the emotional dimension inherent in all painful experiences.

Interpretation of the pain signal is not the result of isolated activity in just one part of the brain. Instead a mosaic of distinct areas of the brain are involved, all interacting closely to "construct" the painful sensation and turn it into something much more than just the detection of a threat. These multiple interactions make pain a very complex perception, strongly influenced by information from several areas of the brain handling emotions, behaviour and awareness. And nothing illustrates this phenomenon better than the dramatic differences in how pain is perceived, depending on the individual and the context surrounding the painful situation.

BEING HARD ON YOUR BODY

Throughout history, doctors have observed that one of the fundamental characteristics of pain is its great variability among individuals, with some people being able to stand discomfort that leaves others exhausted and hopeless. We hear these anecdotes every day — there's the person who continues with his normal activities for several days despite a mild fracture, another who puts off going to the hospital in spite of a long-lasting pain, or a tough guy who doesn't let a persistent headache stop him from using his jackhammer.

Soldiers' injuries clearly illustrate how these individual and sociocultural factors influence pain perception. We have known for a long time that high stress conditions can radically decrease the intensity of pain. For example, if you sprain your ankle, the pain experience will be different depending on whether this injury occurred during your daily jog or while you were trying to escape from a threatening pursuer. It's very likely that the pain will be much less intense if someone is at your heels!

In addition to stressful conditions, the general context in which an injury occurs also influences pain perception. In a now-famous study, a researcher compared the attitude toward pain of 150 soldiers wounded during the allied landing on the beach at Anzio, Italy, with that of 150 civilians of the same age hospitalized following surgery (Beecher, 1946). He observed that even though the soldiers' injuries were more serious, only 32 percent of them expressly asked for painkillers to fight the pain, whereas 83 percent of the civilians wanted them! This difference was due to how the two groups viewed pain: the soldiers viewed their wounds as "positive" since they meant the end of their participation in the fighting and their return home; conversely, the civilians viewed theirs negatively, for they represented a threat to their physical well-being as well as their ability to earn their living. This study revolutionized our approach to pain by shedding light for the first time on the extent to which pain is not just the result of tissue or nerve damage from an injury, but is instead a subjective experience strongly influenced by its context. As a

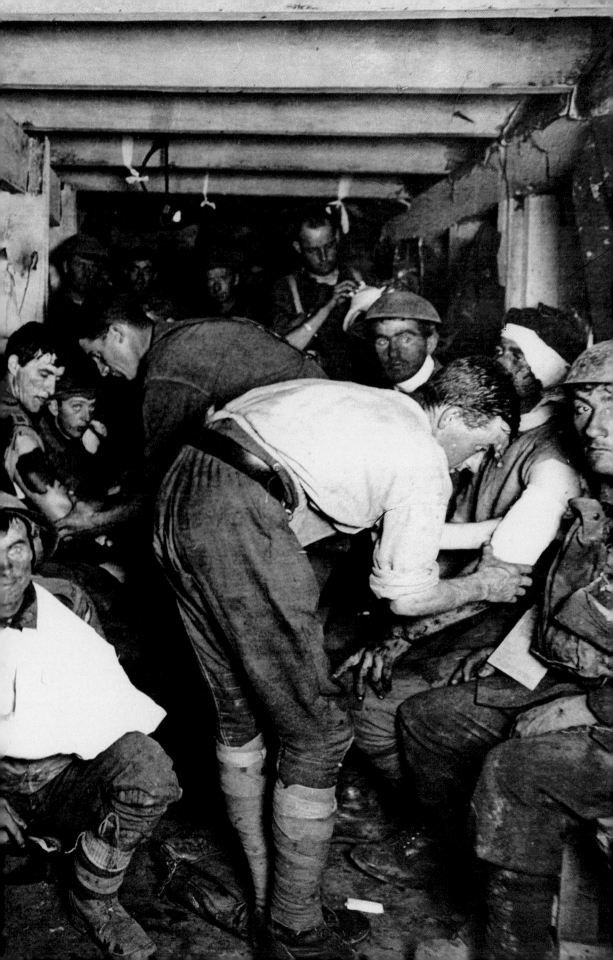

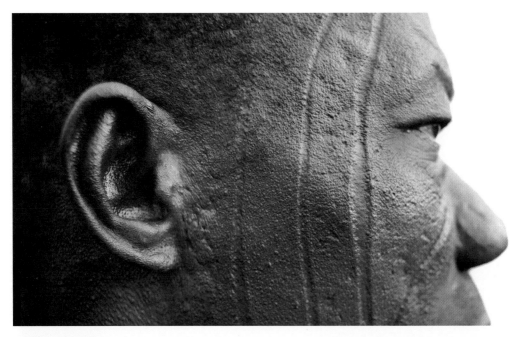

Ritual Pain

In some cultures, rites of passage may consist of extremely demanding physical ordeals. As an example, ethnologists have described the ceremonies celebrating the transition of boys to adulthood in several African peoples, notably the Barabaigs in Tanzania.

In this culture, the boys' hair is first shaved off and three deep incisions are made, sometimes cutting through the skin right to the skull bone, from ear to ear on the face. This kind of rite must certainly be very painful, but the scars (gar) produced by this initiation are displayed with pride by the boys, as the symbol of their new status as men. As with most other documented rites of passage, the pain that accompanies these ordeals is deliberately inflicted to underscore the importance of the transition to adulthood.

Pain is also a part of many religious rites; so-called "redemptive" pain offers a way to communicate with or become closer to the gods. In the Christian religion, for example, pain was once considered to be the most certain way to achieve union with Christ, whether through extreme privation or very severe mortification of the flesh.

In other cultures, pain can be a means of expression intended to obtain favours from the gods. For example, a Tamil ritual to thank the god Murugan (Kârttikeya) involves piercing the skin with sharp steel spikes, or, for the bravest, being suspended in the air for several hours on metal hooks attached to the back of the thighs, calves and shoulder blades. The participants don't appear to feel any pain!

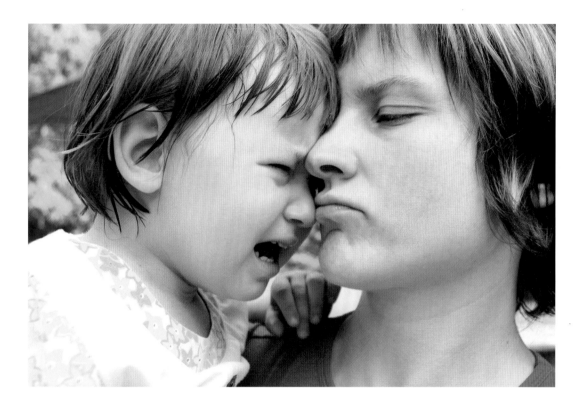

result of these observations, as well as those concerning the exceptional stamina of people who participate in especially challenging routines, it's now recognized that in addition to the activation of the nerve pathways involved in the transmission of a pain signal several psychological factors are equally significant in our assessment of pain. These factors lead us to believe that it's possible to consciously control the signal.

FROM THE BRAIN'S POINT OF VIEW

The preceding examples, including the story of the Italian soldiers, show how much the perception of pain can vary in different cultures and according to the meaning ascribed to the event that causes it. But how can perception vary so much? After all, if the function of pain is to alert the brain to the presence of danger, should this signal not be similarly intense for everyone, regardless of the context of the injury?

In reality, while the primary function of pain is indeed to alert the brain to a threat by transmitting information from the periphery to the control centre ("from bottom to top"), there is another control mechanism that looks closely at the information and adjusts its intensity according to orders issued by the brain: this is the descending pain pathway, which runs from the top down. Let's look again at the analogy of the building security head. While he expects to receive constant reports on the external situation, he nonetheless retains the prerogative to do what he wants with this information. In the case of certain especially strong

Pain's Gatekeeper

Proposed in 1965 by Quebecer Ronald Melzack at McGill University and Englishman Patrick Wall, the "gate control theory of pain" revolutionized our view of the mechanisms that cause pain and still plays a predominant role in a number of approaches designed to treat patients with chronic pain (TENS, medullary stimulation).

From Descartes on (1596–1650), pain had been viewed as a strictly "mechanical" phenomenon, a sensation that stimulated a very specific region of the brain. Melzack and Wall, however, showed that this view could not explain several types of pain, notably phantom limb pain. They therefore theorized that pain might instead be the result of a large number of interactions and exchanges of information occurring at the heart of the nervous system — a "neuromatrix" that analyzes and integrates all pain signals.

This complex theory is based on the premise that the brain is able to "open" or "close" the "gates" the nociceptive signals pass through and can also slow down or speed up the transmission of these signals. It's able to do this by means of a specialized kind of neuron inhibitor — the interneuron — that acts like a gatekeeper and decides how wide to open the gate. In normal circumstances, this neuron is in active mode and secretes endorphins, a class of molecules similar to morphine, putting the pain-causing neurons "to sleep" and reducing their ability to transmit a pain signal. However, when a pain signal is detected on the periphery and relayed to the spinal cord, the gatekeeper is neutralized and the "gate" can swing wide open, immediately allowing the entire pain message to be transmitted to the brain (Figure 15). The goal of pain control mechanisms is therefore to "help" the gatekeeper and give it the chance to begin secreting endorphins again. The endorphins then "close the door," thus reducing the intensity of the pain signal.

Several known physiological, emotional, and cognitive factors can determine the width of the gateway and thus influence the pain's intensity. Adopting lifestyle habits that lessen the influence of negative factors, while making room for positive factors, is a good way to enhance quality of life for people with chronic pain.

nociceptive signals, like those caused by a kidney stone, for example, the brain's interpretation is usually perfectly clear: the signal is perceived as a very serious threat, and the intensity of the pain reaches high levels that are normally very hard to tolerate. On the other hand, most kinds of pain we have to deal with are seldom that intense, and the brain's response to these signals can be much more nuanced. Everyone knows that pain bothers us less when we are busy doing something interesting (reading a good book, watching a movie, holding a conversation); conversely, it can become even harder to tolerate if we focus our attention on it. It's not accidental that parents who have to console children who've hurt themselves use all sorts of tricks to try and make them think about something

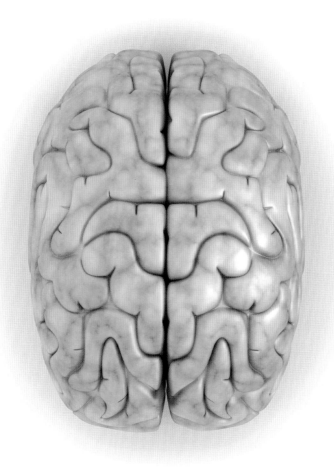

else. In some extreme cases, the brain's influence can even make the difference between life and death. To go back to an example given earlier, the life of an injured person who's trying to run away from an attacker depends largely on how fast he or she can run. In a situation like this, the brain considers the pain from a sprained ankle to be an event of lesser importance compared with the possible consequences of being caught and it therefore tries to reduce the pain's intensity so as not to harm the person's chances of getting away.

Far from being a simple response triggered by an injury, pain is in fact a judgement rendered by the brain as to the danger posed by this injury, an "opinion" that varies depending on the intensity of the pain signal and the context

THE GATE CONTROL THEORY OF PAIN

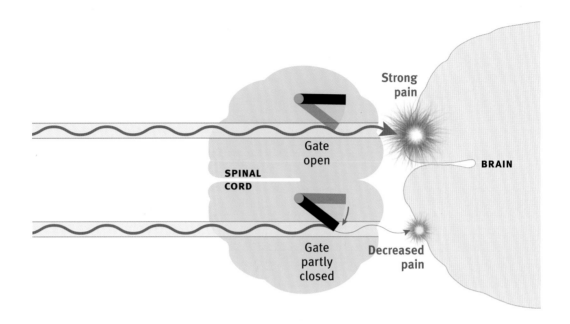

The main factors involved in opening and closing the gate and controlling the intensity of the pain

	Conditions that open the gate (STRONGER PAIN)	Conditions that close the gate (WEAKER PAIN)
PHYSIOLOGICAL	Significant injury or damage	Pharmacological treatment
	Physical inactivity	Stimulation (e.g. massage)
EMOTIONAL	Anxiety	Rest (sleep)
	Depression	Pleasant emotions, optimism, happiness
MENTAL	Focusing on pain	Intense concentration or distraction
	Boredom	Interesting activities

FIGURE 15

in which the pain occurs. If the context makes the pain "positive" or "desirable," as in the case of the wounded soldiers, it's perceived as being much less intense than if it resulted from normal daily activities. In other words, the brain is not just a simple receptor of the pain message: while the pain sensation generated by an injury is identical from one person to another, whatever the circumstances, it's the interpretation of this sensation by the brain that causes the intensity of the pain to vary according to the sociocultural and emotional context at the time of the injury.

CLOSING THE DOOR ON PAIN

These differences in perception are due to specific nerve structures that connect in the opposite direction, "from top to bottom," the various areas in the brain involved in pain perception to certain highly specific parts of the nervous system (the descending pathway) (Figure 14). Our thoughts and emotions are not abstract phenomena occurring "in a vacuum," with no impact on bodily functions. Quite the opposite! What we feel is relayed by the nervous system to our entire organism and influences our physical well-being positively or negatively; it's this close communication between our mental and physical functions that explains, for example, why we lose our appetite when we feel sad or why our heartbeat speeds up in a moment of anger. In the case of pain, the communication network is less obvious but no less essential to the perception of the pain signal. For example, some areas in the brain involved with

thoughts and emotions (the prefrontal cortex and the cingulate anterior cortex, among others) also emit signals that are passed to the brain stem, the most ancient part of our brain (the so-called reptilian brain). There they can interact with slow fibres in the ascending pain pathways to modulate the intensity of the pain message they carry before it reaches the upper brain. Even more importantly, these brain stem structures act as a springboard to relay signals to the spinal cord, where they have a decisive influence on the overall intensity of the pain message.

The strategy used by the descending pathway to alleviate pain is elegant in its simplicity: since pain is caused by too many nociceptive signals, the objective of the control mechanism is to reduce the quantity of these pain signals as much as possible by blocking them right from the start, even before they reach the pathways that carry them to the brain. This is a logical step: after all, the best way to control an event is simply to stop it from happening in the first place!

Since the dorsal root of the spinal cord is the entry point for nerves leading to the central nervous system, this area is the perfect spot for a control system. A good way to visualize how this control system works is to compare it to a system installed on a door to limit certain visitors' access to a house. In the course of evolution, the nervous system developed a series of "gates," small doors that can be opened to varying degrees to control the quantity of nociceptive nerve impulses that manage to reach the brain. These gates are the key to controlling pain, the "gatekeeper" that determines in large part how intensely the pain is felt.

Differences in pain perception, depending on the individual and the context in which the pain occurs, are therefore directly related to the brain's decision as to how wide open the gate should be (Figure 15). An anxious message or an emotional imbalance caused by depression "opens" the gate and heightens the perception of pain. However, a favourable emotional and cognitive climate, such as that found in people who are calm, active, and have an optimistic view of life, "closes" this gate and makes the pain feel less intense.

In addition to these messages from the brain, stimulating the nerve fibres involved in non-painful tactile sensations — touching, rubbing, vibrating — can also close the gate. These sensitive fibres enter the spinal cord along the same pathway as the fibres that transport pain signals; they activate the neurons controlling the opening of the gate and reduce the number of painful nerve impulses that get through. This is the mechanism at work when we instinctively squeeze, rub or shake a sore limb following a painful event, like hitting our thumb with a hammer: by activating the sensory pathways of touch, these instinctive reactions lead to a slight narrowing of the gate so as to limit the entry of nociceptive impulses and thus decrease the perception of pain. In this way, the body can deliberately produce its own "endogenous" analgesia, paving the way for a whole range of interventions designed to alleviate pain.

Pain is much more than just an unpleasant sensation following an injury; it's also the brain's interpretation of this sensation, a perception strongly influenced by the emotional and cognitive processes specific to each person. And this perception has major repercussions on the lives of people in pain.

In Summary

- Pain perception is very complex, involving both physical sensations and a subjective and emotional component.

- All the information needed by the brain to analyze every situation and make a decision, taking into account the context of the information, is transmitted by the nervous system.

- Pain can be controlled by non-painful stimulation of certain areas of the body, by massaging them, for example, and thus alleviating pain.

- Several areas in the brain involved in emotions, behaviour and awareness can influence pain perception by decreasing the intensity of the pain signal.

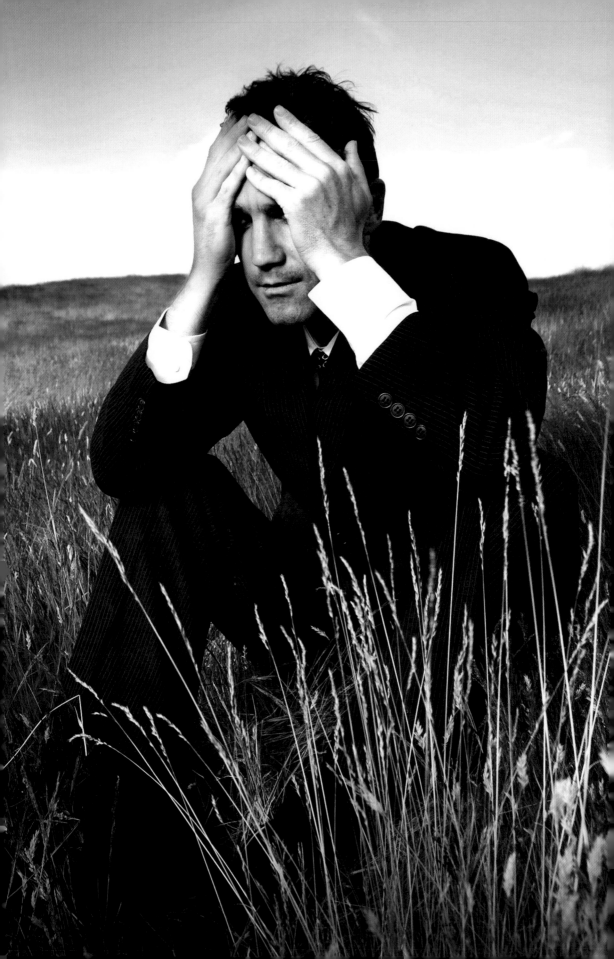

CHAPTER 3

Lives Turned Upside Down

Pleasure is oft a visitant, but pain
Clings cruelly to us.

— JOHN KEATS

The brain's key role in pain perception doesn't mean that your pain is, as people sometimes say, "all in your head." This may seem obvious at first glance, but it's something we have to remember: all pain is real. People suffering from chronic pain sometimes have to put up with hurtful words from those around them — "My brother-in-law had the same problem as you and he went back to work without complaining two days after he got out of the hospital." In addition, they often feel they have to justify their pain, almost as though they have to prove that the pain they're feeling is not imaginary or that they're not exaggerating its impact: "With all the drugs you're taking, it can't be as bad as all that!" This is a frustrating and demoralizing situation for people, especially when the cause of their pain can't be precisely determined or they have to deal with a certain degree of skepticism from medical staff with regard to their situation. If people say they are in pain, we must believe them and not presume to judge their tolerance threshold. This trust is the cornerstone of chronic pain treatment, the foundation that all medical and psychological interventions designed to improve patient outcomes are based on. It's vital to believe that people really are experiencing this pain and to understand that this is a complex phenomenon with both physical and emotional components. The pain's intensity is not so much what the health care professional and family and friends imagine it to be, but rather what the patient says it is.

Keeping this kind of open mind is important, for pain is much more than a disorder in a particular part of the body; the pain felt by people with arthritis does of course originate in their joints, but this pain affects their entire personality and changes every aspect of their lives.

Chronic pain can, in a way, be thought of as an "onion-peel" disease — a multi-dimensional disorder encompassing three major components (Figure 16). To the initial physical sensation (nociception), which activates the nerve pain pathways, is added the brain's interpretation of this sensation (perception), as well as the impact of this interpretation on emotions and behaviour, with each of these factors increasing the burden of chronic pain on quality of life. Pain is a unique experience that's hard to cope with, primarily because it involves the whole person and its disruptions have significant lifestyle repercussions. When you live in pain you are transported to a world where all day-to-day events take on new coloration and you are encumbered by an unrecognizable and unfamiliar body that you have to learn to live with differently.

PAIN AS THE SUM OF PHYSICAL, PSYCHOLOGICAL AND COGNITIVE COMPONENTS

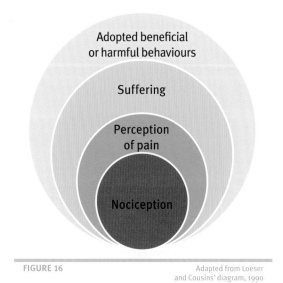

FIGURE 16

Adapted from Loeser
and Cousins' diagram, 1990

DRASTIC LIFESTYLE CHANGES

One of the first effects of chronic pain is to disrupt a way of life to such an extent that sufferers can no longer function normally and have to give up a great many activities. Several studies in various parts of the world indicate that two-thirds of those with persistent pain have to deal with significant limitations in carrying out their everyday activities, with this impact being especially severe in people aged twenty to fifty (Figure 17). All aspects of daily life are touched in varying degrees by pain, whether they be personal (sleep, leisure activities, social relationships) or professional (Figure 18).

While everyone experiences pain differently, it's nonetheless possible to outline the main lifestyle disruptions experienced by the vast majority of patients. These disruptions often trigger actual mourning for losses that are very hard to accept and have a negative influence on morale. And the greater the emotional suffering, the more significant the impacts of pain on day-to-day activities.

DECLINING PHYSICAL ABILITIES AND WORK

People with chronic pain can no longer perform the same physical activities they once did and must, in a way, mourn the loss of their body, since it will never be the same again. This adaptation means calling into question a number of lifestyle habits that rely on the close relationship between the body and the outside world. People who live with pain stop participating in their favourite sports activities first, and in so doing deprive themselves of enjoyable occasions that have long been part of their daily lives. When the pain persists and gets worse, other movements, even harmless ones, are also affected, so that activities as simple as walking, getting out of a chair or even lifting certain light objects can't be done without feeling intense pain. This decline in physical abilities is very hard to bear and it's common for patients to admit, with tears in their eyes, that they have done nothing enjoyable for several weeks. As an example, the daily obstacles faced by this forty-two-year-old woman with intense back pain as the result of a fall are representative of those described by most of the patients who visit a pain clinic and thousands of others who live with pain that keeps them from doing what they want, how they want.

"This accident has turned my life completely upside-down. I can no longer do a fourth of what I used to do, because the pain is too severe. Playing with the children has become impossible and doing my shopping takes an almost superhuman effort.

So forget about going out with my women friends! In fact, I don't see anybody anymore, because I'm always tired: I sleep badly and I feel weak, without energy. Doing minimal housework and preparing meals is hell! I cook and eat a little because I have to and the kids certainly have to eat, but I'm not really hungry and my heart isn't in it."

The pain extends far beyond its specific location; the whole body stiffens up for lack of movement, since the muscles as a whole atrophy and can no longer perform routine movements with ease. Even household chores can become an almost insurmountable obstacle: setting the table, making the bed, or vacuuming, ordinary actions formerly done almost automatically become harder and harder and use up a large amount of energy. Over time, tasks that need to be done regularly are at first done less often and more slowly, and then, in the case of some people, are gradually abandoned.

LIMITATIONS ON DAILY ACTIVITIES IMPOSED BY CHRONIC PAIN

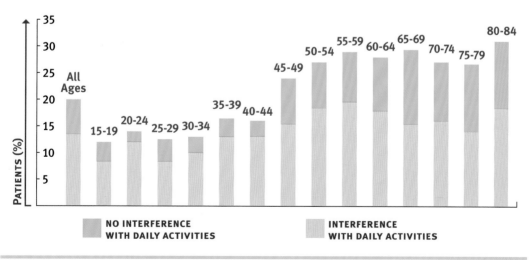

FIGURE 17

Blyth et al., 2001

"I simply can't do the chores I used to do so easily anymore. I can't even unload the dishwasher now! My windows are dirty because I can't raise my arms anymore, there's dust everywhere, my carpets are starting to smell bad … and I used to be such a good housekeeper! Now, I'm ashamed when people come to see me."

People who have to cope daily with persistent pain have trouble accurately assessing their bodies' abilities and what they are actually able to accomplish physically. Under normal circumstances, we have an instinctive awareness of our energy and fatigue levels — a point of reference that allows us to adapt our efforts to our energy reserves. People in pain often lose these points of reference, since pain masks their actual abilities, or what they are able to do.

"I don't recognize my body anymore. On one hand, I no longer have any strength, no energy, but at the same time, I tell myself it's not normal to get so tired doing nothing; so then I "push" myself a bit more; I try to forget that it hurts and pretend there's nothing the matter. But I pay the price for it on the days following and go back to square one, doing nothing, just so I can recover. I don't know any more what

LEVEL OF DISRUPTION OF MOST DAILY ACTIVITIES BY CHRONIC PAIN

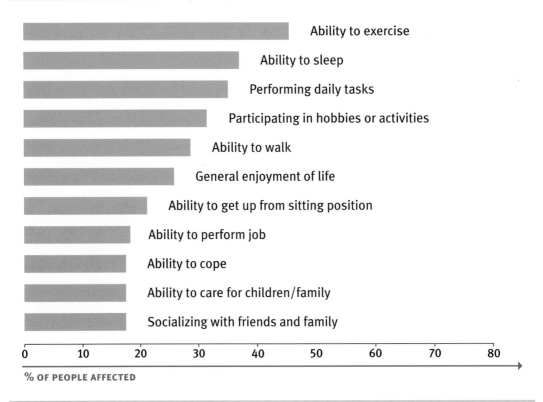

Ability to exercise

Ability to sleep

Performing daily tasks

Participating in hobbies or activities

Ability to walk

General enjoyment of life

Ability to get up from sitting position

Ability to perform job

Ability to cope

Ability to care for children/family

Socializing with friends and family

0   10   20   30   40   50   60   70   80

% OF PEOPLE AFFECTED

FIGURE 18   Lazarus and Neumann, 2001

I can do and what I can't, or how to find a happy medium."

Most people with chronic pain have difficulty figuring out their limits and finding a balance between the energy they have and the energy they use, while at the same time paying attention to the resulting level of pain. At first, people often continue to perform their daily activities in the same way and as intensely as they did before, refusing to accept the decline in their physical abilities. While this is very brave, this kind of approach helps keep the pain at a high level of intensity, as well as causing inflammation in the joints, tendons, or other parts of the body. Despite the individual's best efforts, the body doesn't have the ability to recover enough to recharge its batteries and, after a while, can no longer manage to keep up the pace imposed by what it perceives as too many activities.

The physical impacts of chronic pain also have very negative repercussions on professional activities. This situation is especially unfortunate for manual workers, who need a properly functioning body to carry out daily tasks at work, for carrying heavy loads, doing a job requiring certain repetitive movements, or using tools.

"I worked for seventeen years for this company, lifting and transporting boxes. I was the strongman in the shop! But I hurt myself and I can't push myself like I used to. The bosses were nice to me and transferred me to a job with light work, but I was still in too much pain and had to stop working. My body's worn out and I'm not good for anything anymore. What's going to happen to me?"

In other cases, the work is less physically demanding, and instead it's difficulties

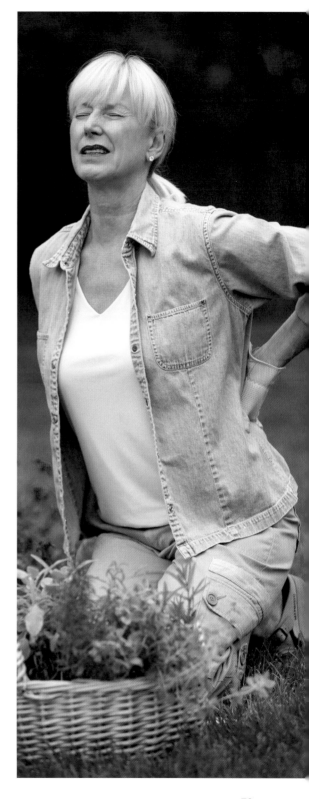

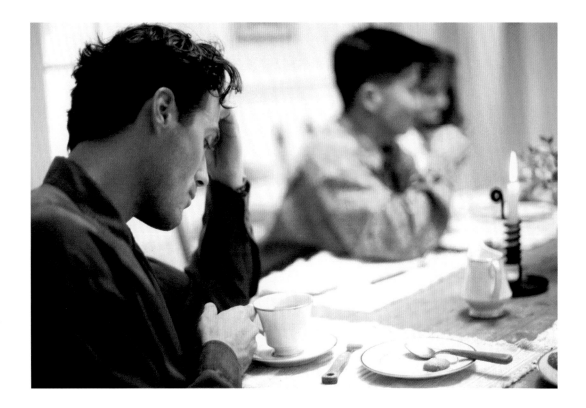

with concentration, attention span, and memory, associated with the pain, medication, or effects on morale, that can cause problems. In time, this can create palpable tension between employees and their colleagues or employers. An experienced receptionist with a painful shoulder told us how she couldn't seem to work, forgot meet-ings, couldn't remember essential information, and often made careless mistakes. These difficulties were closely related to the greater and greater hold that pain had over this woman; she was obliged to remain seated for several hours in a position that was no longer comfortable for her, an ordeal made worse by fatigue caused by a series of nights of poor sleep.

The consequences of this decline in productivity are huge (Figure 19): fewer hours worked and recurring absenteeism,

THE FINANCIAL IMPACTS OF CHRONIC PAIN

Among Canadian adults with chronic pain

Experienced a drop in income because of chronic pain **49%**

Had to reduce their professional responsibilities **47%**

Lost a job because of pain **33%**

FIGURE 19   Canadian Pain Survey,
                    The Canadian Pain Society, 2007

as well as a reduced workload, mean a decline in income for nearly half of chronic pain sufferers. Short- or medium-term temporary leave from work or an extended absence of indeterminate length are of course an option, but compensation packages are often not very well suited to the realities of people with chronic pain and can cause insurance problems. All these factors help create a feeling of helplessness and anxiety in many people living with pain; this can lead to emotional fatigue and a drop in the energy they need to look after themselves. In a third of workers, the stress caused by declining efficiency has more extreme consequences that can lead to early retirement, being fired, or resigning.

By doing away with the usual points of reference, the markers that enable people to get their bearings and navigate through life, chronic pain can become a synonym for failure, an apparently insurmountable obstacle to carrying out our projects and achieving our ambitions. Few events lead us to question ourselves as fundamentally as chronic pain, since it forces sufferers to redefine their life goals to adjust to this new reality.

SLEEP

Of all our daily activities, sleep has the most underestimated positive impact on our health. Sleeping well lets us replenish our body's energy reserves, consolidate what we have learned (the saying "sleep on it" actually does have a biochemical and neurological basis), and plays a key role in stabilizing emotions and in our psychological well-being.

Quality of sleep is directly related to the situations and emotions people experience during the day. Intense stress or an especially happy or exciting event can shorten sleep time, while on the other hand an exhausting day of work is followed by a longer period of sleep. These variations are normal and have no negative effect on health. Sleep time returns to normal over the following nights, so we can regain the balance needed for physical and emotional well-being.

Sleep disturbances are among the main kinds of collateral damage caused by chronic pain, and they play a leading role in the deterioration in quality of life of sufferers. Much scientific research on the connection between pain and sleep shows that most patients with chronic pain have sleep problems — trouble getting to sleep and staying asleep, waking up too early, sleep that isn't restorative, and fatigue (Figure 21). This lack of sleep is often felt by sufferers to be as important as their pain.

THE SLEEP/PAIN CYCLE

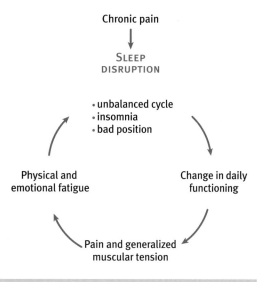

FIGURE 20

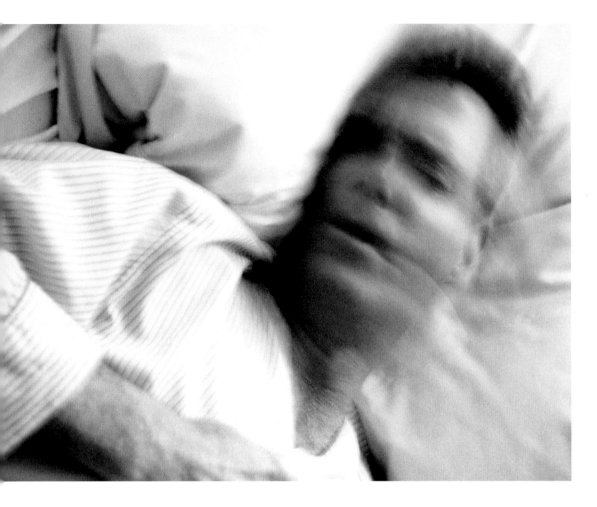

SLEEP DISTURBANCES (INSOMNIA) IN PEOPLE WITH CHRONIC PAIN

Sleep-related characteristics

Difficulty initiating sleep 43 %

Disrupted sleep 43 %

Early morning awakenings 44 %

Non-restorative sleep 42 %

Dissatisfaction with quality of sleep 45 %

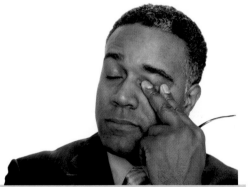

FIGURE 21

Ohayon, 2005

Depression, anxiety, or fatigue, as well as being in poor physical shape, can also contribute to this disruption.

For these people, actually getting to sleep in a reasonable time can be a major challenge; how can you find a comfortable position that lets you drift off to sleep when your body is in a more or less permanent state of tension and discomfort? Often they have to spend several hours trying to find a minimum of comfort, constantly changing position or the number and arrangement of pillows before managing to fall asleep, frequently from exhaustion. Once a special time of day to look forward to, sleep becomes a dreaded ordeal approached with anxiety. Other people manage to fall asleep quickly but are awakened a few hours later by persistent tension and discomfort and can't get back to sleep. This situation is hardly any better, since the hours of insomnia that follow, which we are mercilessly reminded of when we glance at our alarm clock, causes stress that makes falling asleep again even harder.

Having trouble getting a good night's sleep results in an imbalance in the normal sleep-wake cycle that can accelerate the deterioration in quality of life associated with chronic pain. One problem is that not getting truly restorative sleep results in accumulated fatigue and therefore makes it more difficult to carry out normal daily tasks. Furthermore, sleep deprivation also modifies pain perception mechanisms, making the pain more intense (Lautenbacher et al., 2006). Disturbed sleep thus drags the sufferer into another damaging vicious circle where lack of sleep leads to greater fatigue, and this fatigue in turn increases the intensity

Stephen, 35

For several years, Stephen has suffered from persistent headaches. These migraines can occur at any time, but they become especially incapacitating when there are other people around: the cacophony of many competing conversations makes the intensity of the pain unbearable. So as not to find himself in these difficult situations, Stephen now avoids public places and no longer even goes to gatherings organized by his and his spouse's families. These repeated absences have cast a serious chill over his family relationships, a situation his spouse, for whom these events are extremely important, finds very hard to accept. Nor can she invite her family over to their house like she used to and, on the rare occasions when they do come to visit, Stephen retreats to his workshop to avoid making his migraines worse.

Susan, 51

Susan has had fibromyalgia for many years. She has become hypersensitive to any kind of physical contact, no matter how slight, and now finds her spouse's touch unpleasant and aggressive. He doesn't know how to approach her physically, afraid to hurt her and be rejected again. The two are growing apart and it's causing them great unhappiness.

of the pain — which then disrupts sleep even more (Figure 20).

The physical fatigue caused by a lack of sleep is inevitably accompanied by emotional fatigue. People who can no longer sleep well are often depressed, sad, and discouraged, and may over time develop anxiety and depression disorders. The pain-sleep-depression triad is in fact a fundamental characteristic of chronic pain. Everyone with chronic pain must therefore pay special attention to the quality of their sleep, for it's impossible to properly treat persistent pain without assessing and treating a possible sleep problem.

DIET

Most people with chronic pain mention major changes in their eating habits and these changes almost always mean a decline in the quality of their diet. Obviously, this situation stems largely from the physical constraints pain imposes: these people simply don't have enough energy to get out to shop, make the necessary efforts to keep food constantly in stock and prepare tasty well-balanced meals, especially if the pain is accompanied by a drop in income, forcing people to make choices about the quantity and quality of food. What often ensues is a growing lack of interest in anything to do with food — either cooking it or eating it. Some people experience a noticeable loss of appetite, which may be made worse by the side effects of medication (loss of sense of taste, constipation, diarrhea) or psychological distress (depression). In others, one way of getting around the difficulty of shopping and cooking is to eat only readily available processed food, despite the fact that these are usually lower quality foods with high levels of sugar, salt, and bad fats. The high caloric intake associated with eating this kind of food can also, over time, result in weight gain, especially when people eat out of boredom or because they are feeling down.

The impact of these changes on the well-being of people with chronic pain must not be underestimated. Food is our fuel, the source of the energy our bodies need to function, and any imbalance in the type or quality of diet can't help but have harmful consequences. In addition, it's frequently noted that the physical exhaustion typical of people with chronic pain is caused as much by dietary deficiencies as by the pain itself. Conversely, overweight caused by a poor quality high-calorie diet lacking in nutrients can lead to pain in the knee joints, legs, and lower back, disrupt sleep, and have a negative impact on self-image and self-esteem. All of these outcomes are negative. People who are poorly nourished will have trouble dealing with their pain, since dietary deficiencies cause an energy or nutrient deficiency that makes the burden of the pain even harder to bear.

DETERIORATING SOCIAL, FAMILY, AND COUPLES RELATIONSHIPS

In addition to personal hardship, declining physical abilities, and the fatigue felt by people with chronic pain also changes their relationships with those close to them and their social life in general. Leisure activities, formerly pleasant occasions for meeting friends, are often the first activities to suffer because the person has no energy, and opportunities to socialize quickly become less and less frequent. And even when they do take place, these

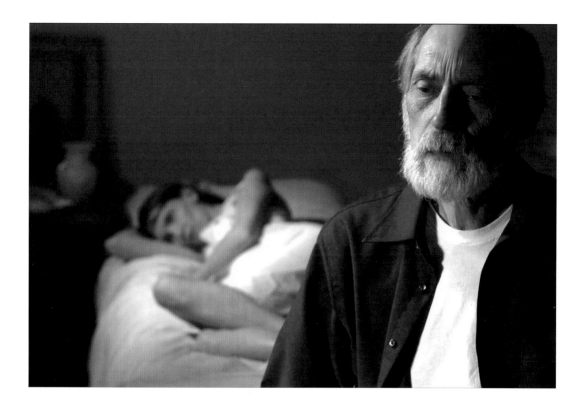

events are not quite as enjoyable as before, since the conversations invariably revolve around the person's pain, its impacts on day-to-day life, doctor's visits, etc. After a while, these occasions occur less and less often for want of new events that might be of common interest and, eventually, friendships that can't adapt to this new reality fade away by themselves.

Spousal relationships can also be sorely tested when one of the partners is dealing with persistent pain. In day-to-day life, tasks have to be shared differently, with the healthy partner having to take on twice as much in an attempt to make up for the other's declining physical abilities. This increasing workload is usually accepted eagerly in the short term, but it sometimes becomes a source of conflicts in the longer term. For example,

the partner who, in addition to working, takes care of all the family's activities outside the home (taking the children to day-care and their activities, doing the grocery shopping, and looking after the yard and the house, as well as car repairs) may expect that meals and housework will be done by the spouse who stays home; this is obviously not always the case, given the spouse's state of health. In the long term, this kind of situation can result in a noticeable deterioration in the couple's relationship, especially since the pain is invisible and the healthy partner may have trouble understanding the other's physical limitations.

Pain also has a major influence on intimate and sexual relations: a touch or a simple caress can cause severe pain, thus making it difficult to find a position comfortable enough for longer periods of intimacy. Fatigue, medications, depression, or anxiety can also cause dysfunction (loss of desire, libido, impotence), going so far as to eliminate sexual relations entirely. In some cases, a deterioration in the physical relationship is the prelude to the partners' growing further and further apart, and the lack of communication and closeness only makes the feelings of frustration, rebellion, or discouragement associated with the pain even stronger.

Erosion of the social fabric is an especially cruel consequence of chronic pain. Faced with the loss of their friends, becoming distant from their spouse, or the impossibility of spending time with their children, people may feel more and more uninteresting and useless, and therefore try to limit interactions with those around them as much as possible: they stay at home, sometimes choosing to shut themselves into one room to avoid any form of contact. This isolation can result in withdrawal from the outside world: they become more and more reluctant to communicate their thoughts and feelings and are less and less inclined to be interested in those of others. Like a cancer whose metastases have invaded the entire organism, pain takes over every aspect of their life.

While pain is first and foremost a physical ordeal, the many obstacles people in pain have to face prevent them from realizing their full potential socially and professionally, thus contributing to the deterioration in their quality of life and self-esteem. These kinds of upheavals are not limited to people who have to face chronic pain daily; to varying degrees, all serious illnesses have an effect on physical and emotional equilibrium and place a heavy burden on patients. Chronic pain, however, is in a class of its own, because negative emotions are not just a result of a physical malfunction, but are really major players in the way this illness is perceived by those affected. And they can become so powerful that they risk dragging sufferers into a downward spiral that it can be difficult to get out of.

In Summary

- Along with chronic pain go many disruptions in daily activities, especially in terms of physical ability and relationships with other people.

- One of the aspects of daily life most disrupted by chronic pain is sleep. A vicious circle takes hold: pain disrupts the quality of sleep, and the fatigue caused by a bad night magnifies the perception of pain.

- All of these upheavals are really bereavements, challenges that are very hard to overcome and that have a negative influence on the emotional balance of those in pain and their quality of life.

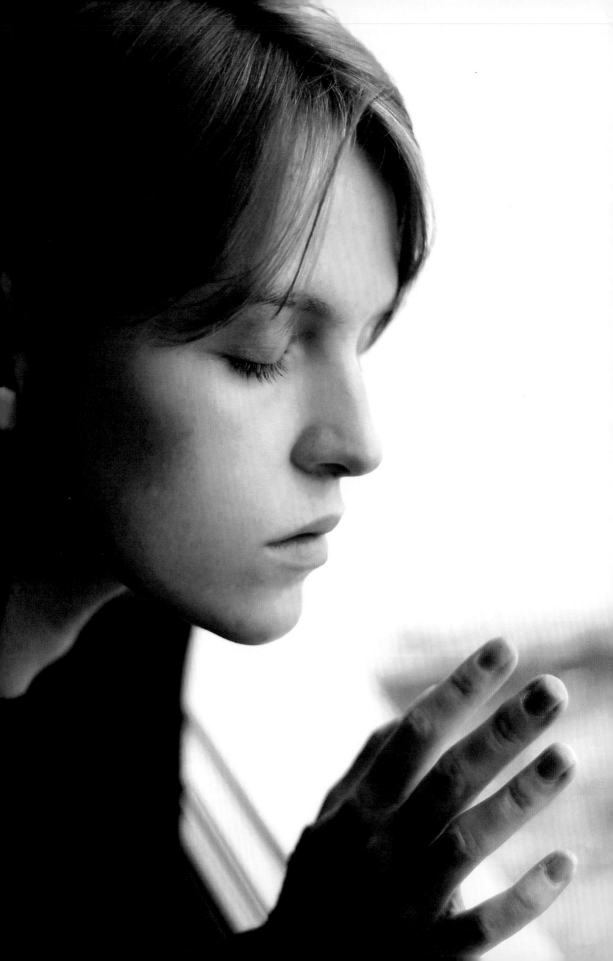

CHAPTER 4

When Emotions Enter the Picture

That's what pain is like, it chockes, it needs more air
Pain needs space.

— MARGUERITE DURAS

It's natural for us to think of the diseases we get as being purely physical attacks, whose negative impact on health is due only to a disruption in the way an organ or a particular biological system functions. However, the body isn't just a bunch of parts all working independently; the cells are constantly listening to each other and exchanging information in the form of molecular signals that allow them to accurately "read" the body's overall condition. This cellular "social network" is a very effective system, ensuring that any imbalance, even if it's localized, is felt throughout the organism. And we often forget that the brain is also part of this communication network: our way of thinking, our emotions or certain reactions like stress are strongly influenced by events occurring in the rest of the body, just as a disruption in neurophysiological processes can also lead to the development of certain diseases.

Good health is the reflection of a healthy mind in a healthy body, with each influencing the other to ensure the harmonious functioning of the organism.

The importance of the body-mind equilibrium is especially well illustrated by the changes that occur in the lives of those dealing with chronic pain. All health professionals who work with these patients come face to face with the enormous psychological distress that's so much a part of pain: the sufferers' words echo through their offices.

A WINDOW ON THE SOUL

Very broadly speaking, emotion can be defined as a spontaneous change in our state of mind in response to influences in our environment or biochemical changes in our bodies. Emotions are sometimes pleasant, sometimes unpleasant, but they are always "sincere," that is, they express in a tangible way what we really feel in a particular situation. There are therefore no "good" or "bad" emotions, but simply real emotions corresponding to our state of mind. Although they are still too often viewed as a sign that a person is too sensitive, and sometimes even as a sign of weakness, emotions are actually vitally important, because they are a window on our soul and on how we interpret what happens to us.

This doesn't mean, however, that all emotions are compatible with good mental and physical health! In some circumstances, notably in cases of chronic pain, emotions that cause distress, like anxiety, sadness, or anger, can contribute dramatically to the burden of the illness. It's therefore important to better understand the factors controlling emotions, so as to reduce their harmful influence and enhance the quality of life of people in pain.

Emotion is a complex experience with both psychological and physiological components. On the one hand, research conducted using magnetic resonance imaging has shown that a very specific region in the brain, the limbic system, plays a predominant role in emotions and feelings (Figure 22). Located in the centre of the brain, this system comprises the amygdala, the anterior cingulate cortex, and the hippocampus. These three regions are closely connected to other parts of the brain, especially the cortex responsible for cognitive abilities. As a result, the emotions generated by the limbic system influence the way we think, just as the cognitive processes stemming from activity in the cortex can have an

effect on emotions. The impact of emotions on pain perception is clearly shown in the results of imaging studies. By examining carefully the activation of areas of the brain involved in pain perception using functional magnetic resonance imaging, researchers have shown that negative or positive emotions had an influence on activity in these regions and, as a result, on the intensity with which the pain was perceived (Roy et al., 2009).

On the other hand, emotion triggers many physiological effects that directly influence an individual's behaviour: increased heart rate, secretion of certain hormones, changes in muscular function. These changes in turn cause the physical symptoms associated with emotions: trembling, pallor or redness, facial expressions, changes in bowel habits. Thoughts, emotions, and behaviours thus interact constantly and influence each other, with a very significant impact on our well-being.

OUR THOUGHTS

When we are faced with a particular situation, the assessment we make using our cognitive abilities (our thoughts) is the main cause of the emotions we feel and the behaviours we adopt in this situation (Figure 23). A good example of the positive aspect of these interactions is the pleasure and excitement people feel on hearing a melody they especially like: happy thoughts triggered by listening to the song give rise to an emotion (joy) which, in turn, influences the body (shivers) and behaviour (singing or dancing). This influence is not one-way: emotions and physiological states

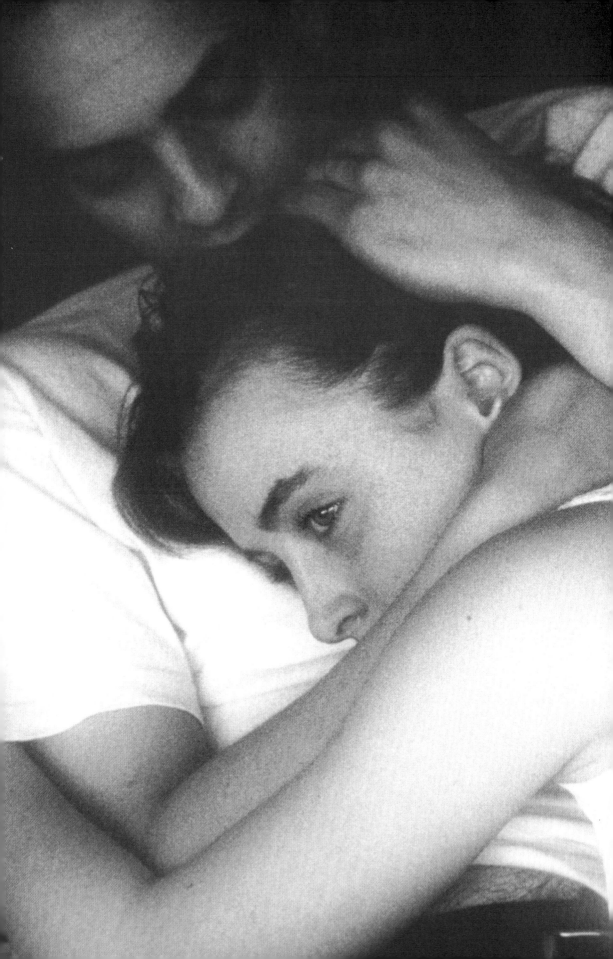

also influence thoughts; this means that our physical state can determine in large part how we interpret an event. For example, if this same person broke a leg a few days earlier, is in pain and has had trouble getting around since then, it's unlikely that the song will trigger happy thoughts or great joy, let alone the urge to dance!

In the case of chronic pain, thoughts are often harmful, since sufferers will view the pain mainly from the perspective of what has been lost, the limits imposed, and the pain to be tolerated. Individuals in pain may say to themselves from the moment they wake up: "It still hurts, if only I couldn't feel the pain for a few seconds. What have I done that I should suffer like this?" A series of thoughts like this, understandable but nonetheless "black," obviously has a direct impact on people's behaviour and emotions and can't help but have an impact on all the activities that they later have to accomplish.

The influence of these thoughts is not always easy to determine. For example, someone may feel sad for no apparent reason or be suddenly struck by a panic attack while preparing a meal or right in the middle of the night, without any specific situation or thought being able to explain this anxiety. But, in reality, this isn't quite the case. Thoughts arise from people's assessment of a situation, from what they tell themselves about what's going on around them. These thoughts are very often unconscious and therefore harder to identify, but they still have lasting personal repercussions.

THE LIMBIC SYSTEM

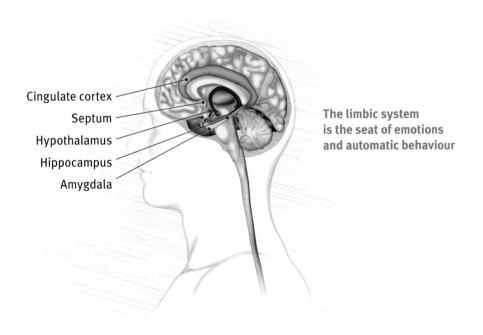

Cingulate cortex
Septum
Hypothalamus
Hippocampus
Amygdala

The limbic system is the seat of emotions and automatic behaviour

FIGURE 22   Adapted from *Les thérapies comportementales et cognitives (Behavioural and Cognitive Therapies)*, First Éditions

The example of Jane helps us to fully understand the power of thoughts, even when they are buried deep in our minds and we only become aware of them after much reflection. These deeper thoughts, which often dictate our actions and behaviours, are called beliefs. Psychologically speaking, beliefs are people's fundamental ideas about themselves, their experiences, and their relationships with the world around them. Some beliefs take root in childhood, while others develop after traumatic events or major life changes, like the onset of chronic pain. What we observe in such cases is a fundamentally negative narrative, showing how difficult it is for people to face up to the situation they find themselves in (Figure 24).

Fundamentally negative beliefs about pain and people living with it take an "all or nothing" approach; the underlying thoughts focus only on losses, whether real or perceived, and on the fears and disappointments related to the pain, without considering some of its more positive aspects, like support from family and friends. Beliefs may also reflect the potential dangers associated with pain and discomfort, including the fear of not finding relief from the pain, feeling even more pain and getting hurt again, having to give up our career, or being rejected or abandoned by those around us.

So it's not really the pain as such that triggers emotions, but rather our thoughts, what we tell ourselves consciously or unconsciously when we think about the pain. Indeed, several studies indicate

THE THOUGHTS-EMOTIONS-BEHAVIOURS TRIAD

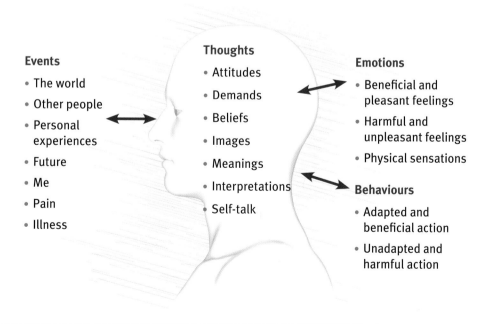

Events
- The world
- Other people
- Personal experiences
- Future
- Me
- Pain
- Illness

Thoughts
- Attitudes
- Demands
- Beliefs
- Images
- Meanings
- Interpretations
- Self-talk

Emotions
- Beneficial and pleasant feelings
- Harmful and unpleasant feelings
- Physical sensations

Behaviours
- Adapted and beneficial action
- Unadapted and harmful action

FIGURE 23   Adapted from *Les thérapies comportementales et cognitives (Behavioural and Cognitive Therapies)*, First Éditions

Jane, 29

Jane is afraid of the dark and panics the minute she finds herself in a dark room. This problem arose recently, after a serious car accident that left her with back and neck pain, extreme fatigue, and trouble sleeping. After talking about it with her psychologist, Jane was able to pinpoint the cause of her anxiety: she was afraid of the dark because she couldn't see anything, didn't know where she was, and therefore felt she was losing control of herself, just like during the car accident. Jane had always prided herself on her self-control and couldn't imagine losing this ability.

that this combination of emotions and thoughts is the main reason behind individual differences in pain perception and the way pain changes people's quality of life. Chronic pain is a complex phenomenon; its interpretation by the brain can be greatly influenced by our emotional and cognitive processes. Successfully adapting to pain therefore means finding a way to modify this self-talk — the "little voice" that tells us what attitude to take when facing a difficult situation, and constantly feeds into this negative feedback loop.

EXAMPLES OF THOUGHTS AND THEIR UNDERLYING BELIEFS

Everyday thoughts, frequently repeated (conscious or not)	Fundamental beliefs (underlie everyday thoughts)
I can't do the vacuuming — what am I good for?	I'm useless
There's nothing I can do to control my pain.	I'm powerless.
I can't ski anymore; it was my whole life.	I can't do anything worthwhile anymore.
Pain is ruining my life.	My life is over.
I can't go to see my kids play soccer anymore; I'm a coward	I'm not a good mother anymore.
I don't have anything interesting to say anymore, because I don't do anything!	I'm not the person I was; I'm not worth much.

FIGURE 24

A ROLLER COASTER RIDE

As in all of life's difficult moments — bereavement, divorce, illness, professional failure — the reactions and emotions caused by chronic pain vary a great deal, depending on how much time has elapsed since the triggering event. While each kind of pain is experienced differently depending on the individual and the sociocultural context of the pain, all emotional and cognitive reactions can nonetheless be divided into two main phases, both of which have a decisive influence on how the pain is perceived and how well people are able to manage its impact on their daily lives (Figure 25). In the first or "descending" phase, sufferers experience a broad range of emotions stemming from the deterioration in their quality of life and the many difficulties imposed by persistent pain. In addition to the initial shock, often severe in the case of violent trauma, this phase is usually accompanied by fear, anger, shame,

guilt, and anxiety, with all of these emotions helping to create a climate of sorrow and despair that can in many cases lead to depression. In turn, these emotions influence how people in pain think and can thus have a considerable effect on their ability to cope with the difficult situation they find themselves in.

This "dark phase" is not irreversible, however. As we will see in detail in the following chapters, people with chronic pain can gradually regain a better quality of life by taking a different approach to their pain, one based not just on medical treatments, but also on changing how they cope cognitively with pain. To do this, we have to understand the extent to which chronic pain upsets people's psychological and emotional defense systems and undermines them by stirring up insecurities that were formerly well under control and gave them stability. These insecurities can turn into a destructive force when they come to the surface and take centre stage.

THE CURVE OF CHRONIC PAIN EMOTIONS

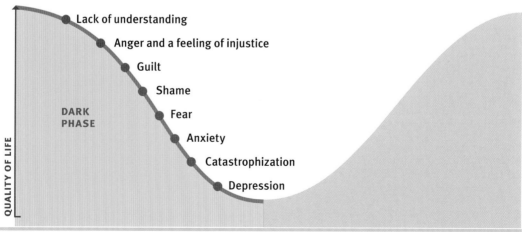

FIGURE 25

Adapted from Couture, 2010

EMOTIONS ACCOMPANYING CHRONIC PAIN

The following emotions are frequently experienced: difficulty understanding, anger, and a sense of injustice, guilt, shame, fear, anxiety, catastrophizing, and depression.

DIFFICULTY UNDERSTANDING

The tragic events that happen to us usually strike without warning, forcing us to react quickly to cope with the upheavals they cause. Pain is no exception to this rule: Whether it's the result of injury or trauma, the onset of a painful sensation always comes as a shock that occurs suddenly and instantly changes the way the body works and its relationship with the outside world. In a situation like this, our first reaction is to consult a doctor as quickly as possible to get treatment that will make the pain go away. At this stage, there's absolutely no reason to think that the situation can't be controlled. When initial treatments prove not very effective and the pain becomes persistent or more intense in the weeks and months that follow, disbelief gives way to growing worry, and then to powerful emotions that can completely change people's lives and the way they inter-act with those around them. Not everyone feels these emotions in the same order, and some may be felt more intensely than others. Thus, one person may feel anger more than anything else right from the onset of pain and stay that way until he or she falls into a depression, whereas for someone else, fear may be the central emotion, with other emotions revolving around it, although the individual may not necessarily be depressed.

ANGER AND PERCEIVED INJUSTICE

As hope for a rapid cure fades with the passing months, people feel very disappointed that the pain is still there and seems to resist various treatment options. With time, these disappointments accumulate and gradually turn into anger, for example, at the circumstances of the accident that caused the pain, at the waiting time to get to see a health care professional, at themselves for not having known how to react at the beginning or for having ignored certain signs. People can even become hostile, aggressive or irritable and react disproportionately to innocuous or unimportant situations. All of these forms of anger indicate frustration at a situation that continues to go downhill and may jeopardize the pleasures of everyday life and future projects — travel, retirement.

"Why me?" is one of the questions that most haunts the minds of people who have seen their lives change dramatically following the onset of chronic pain. Most of the time, this feeling of injustice is the expression of deep distress, of rebellion against a cruel and undeserved fate. This is a normal reaction in the short-term, but it can nonetheless become unhealthy if it goes on too long.

GUILT

Although the factors causing the onset of chronic pain are usually hard to control, people in pain may feel guilty about their situation and the impact it's having on those around them. Having become, in spite of themselves, the centre of other people's attention, they often feel guilty about the many adaptations their family and friends have to make to deal with their state of health: their spouse's responsibilities increase, they play with their children less often, and outings or holiday plans are cancelled at the last minute for fear of a pain crisis.

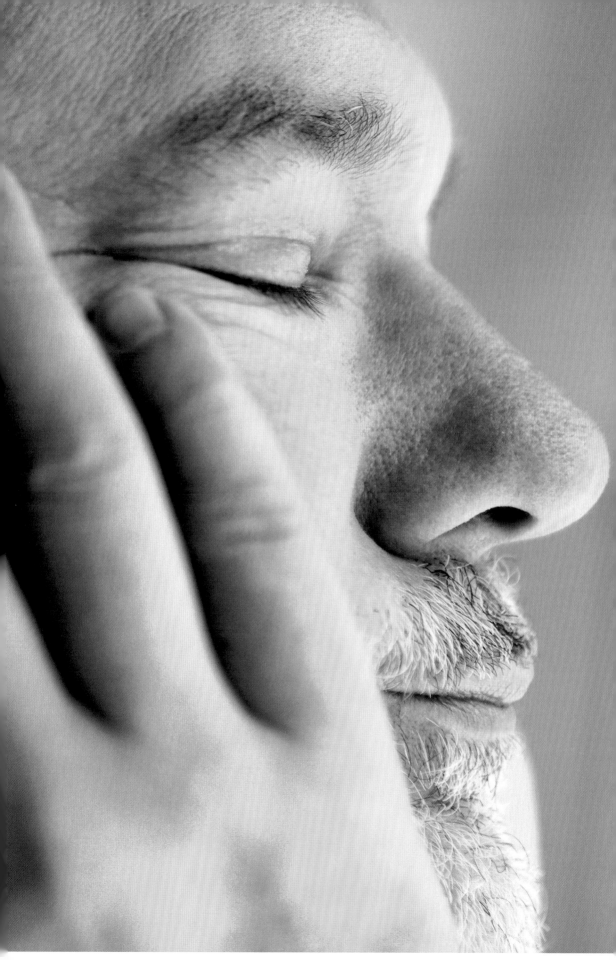

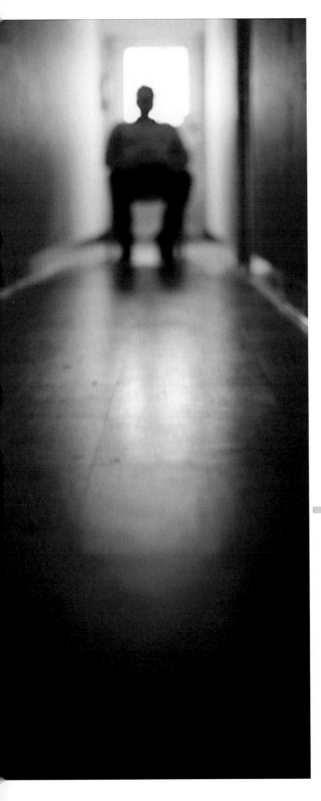

SHAME

Learning to cope with weakened physical abilities is always hard. For some people, this difficulty can become a source of great embarrassment and even shame. These feelings can also be aggravated by the culture of our modern society, in which performance and self-fulfilment have become fundamental values essential for personal and social success, especially when people define themselves by what they do and not by who they are. In this kind of context, people often feel marginalized and lose their self-esteem, suddenly ashamed to no longer be able to contribute the way they once did to their family and to society, for example after losing their job. Dependence on drugs, on disability or social insurance payments, or on food banks for basic necessities are all factors that can perpetuate the shame they feel at having to live with diminished abilities and on the fringes of productive society.

John, 59

A construction worker for over twenty years, John tripped over tools that had not been stowed away properly and injured his legs. He was alone and unable to move for thirty minutes before a co-worker noticed him and came to help. Since then, John's legs hurt a great deal and he's had to quit work, but he feels especially angry at his co-workers, who hadn't put their equipment away correctly. His anger can also be seen in his difficulty in adapting to the new situation: John is convinced the accident should never have happened and that he's the only victim.

FEAR

Fear is a totally understandable reaction for people in pain. When it's excessive, however, fear takes over and throws them off balance, turning pain into their main preoccupation; it takes centre stage in their lives and largely tells them how to think and interact with their environment. This unhealthy control makes the impact of chronic pain even greater, from both the physical and psychological point of view.

Fear of movement — kinesiophobia — is the fear most closely associated with chronic pain, especially when the pain is musculoskeletal. This fear leads people to stay inactive instead of testing their body's ability to accomplish an activity, however simple it may be: they have a tendency to seek reasons not to move, not realizing that their inactivity is linked to their fear of injuring themselves again or increasing the pain. In many cases, therefore, it's not so much the pain that keeps people from moving as the anticipation of pain, the fear of hurting themselves while performing a particular activity.

This fear of movement often makes it possible to feel better in the short term, which, in a way, validates the inactive approach. But this behaviour can become very hard to reverse, for by becoming more and more inactive, people have fewer and fewer opportunities to test their actual physical condition and discover the true intensity of the pain associated with a particular activity. People who stop performing certain tasks, vacuuming, for example, for fear of feeling pain again, may also stop performing other activities they really enjoy (gardening, walks in the woods) and that are not necessarily painful, or that they could tolerate if they began to do them gradually, so as to let their body (and the

Paul, 27

Paul injured his knee badly when he fell skiing. After several operations and many physiotherapy sessions, he resigned himself, sadly, to giving up skiing. Formerly very active and in great physical shape, he also stopped performing most of his daily activities, because he doesn't think he can do them anymore. Paul isn't aware of it, but the fact is that he's scared. He's afraid of making his knee injury worse and causing himself more pain. His fears are perfectly normal, but they are keeping him from achieving his life goals and resuming a more active lifestyle, even if it can't be quite as intense as it was before the accident.

WHEN FEAR CAUSES PAIN AND DISABILITY

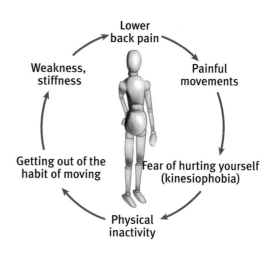

FIGURE 26

99

A Panic Attack

Someone anxious may experience panic attacks along with a series of physical symptoms and thoughts that fuel both the panic itself and anxiety. The Diagnostic and Statistical Manual of Mental Disorders (the DSM-IV) defines a panic attack as a discrete period of intense conscious or unconscious fear or physical discomfort, in which four (or more) of the following symptoms develop abruptly and reach a peak within ten minutes:

1. Palpitations, pounding heart, or accelerated heart rate
2. Sweating
3. Trembling or shaking
4. Sensations of shortness of breath or smothering
5. Feeling of choking
6. Chest pain or discomfort, like a heavy weight on the chest
7. Nausea and abdominal or intestinal distress
8. Feeling dizzy, unsteady, light-headed, or faint
9. Derealization (feelings of unreality) or depersonalization (as if you could watch yourself doing something, with the sensation of being detached from your body)
10. Fear of losing control or going crazy
11. Fear of dying
12. Numbness or tingling sensations in the extremities (fingers, toes, hands, feet)
13. Chills or hot flashes

A panic attack accompanied by several of these symptoms may occur suddenly without any single obvious cause to explain these reactions. In other cases, it can be triggered by a very specific event. Panic can occur, for example, in someone who suffers from agoraphobia, a fear of not being able to get away from a public space; in the medium and long term this can greatly limit outings and result in withdrawal from the outside world.

pain) adapt. Over time, this fear of movement becomes self-sustaining; the avoidance of any potentially painful situation increases their fear of hurting themselves, regardless of the physical activity.

In the long term, this kind of behaviour becomes very detrimental to the body. When there are fewer demands on the muscles, they eventually atrophy and become less able to fulfill their primary function. Over time, this deconditioning of the muscle structure leads to muscular weakness and stiffness that, in turn, causes increased pain during movement. The body gets "stuck" in a vicious circle — pain keeps it from functioning like it used to, resulting in much less movement, and this in itself makes the initial pain worse (Figure 26).

ANXIETY

In contrast to fear, a response to a real and current danger, anxiety is the result of our ability to foresee negative events that could happen in the future. Anxiety is a perception, an assessment of a situation that involves our way of thinking, as well as our confidence in our ability to manage the situation appropriately. In a chronic pain context, it's normal for this way of thinking and this confidence to be sorely tested and for people to develop anxiety given the many changes they face. This anxiety is first and foremost an emotional state, but it can also lead to very troubling physical symptoms (heart palpitations, sweating, shaking, feelings of vertigo, dizzy spells, hot flashes) that in some cases occur suddenly in the form of a panic attack. Anxiety is thus an eloquent example of the close connection between emotions and the body's functioning.

The circumstances surrounding the onset of pain may have been traumatizing, causing patients to develop severe anxiety disorders, such as post-traumatic stress disorder (PTSD). Anxiety is not, however, just a result of trauma. It can reach disproportionate levels in relation to most kinds of pain; in every case this makes it impossible for people to take a more constructive approach to the problem and draw on their inner resources to find ways to cope with it. This kind of extreme anxiety is frequently observed in patients whose pain has become their main preoccupation, the centre of their lives around which all their thoughts and emotions revolve. This inordinate amount of attention means that patients see all the situations they face as threats. Anxiety can reach extreme levels when, at the same time, these patients acquire a tendency toward catastrophizing, constantly imagining the worst possible scenario. This anxiety increases the intensity of the pain and makes treatments less effective or even simply impossible to put into practice.

Jason, 42

One winter's night, Jason was driving on an extremely snowy highway when his car skidded. The paramedics found him with his feet stuck under the pedals and in total shock, his head having violently struck the steering wheel. At the time, Jason complained of searing pain in his feet, back, and neck. Eight months later, a sharp pain in his back still keeps him from walking normally, and he remains very fearful: he hasn't driven a car since the accident and he has become hypervigilant when someone else is driving or he's out walking. He often has nightmares about the accident, and when he hears an ambulance siren he gets tense, begins to sweat, and feels nervous. The fear of death he felt comes back to haunt him, especially the fear of never seeing his two young children again. His partner has noticed he's more distant toward them and that he isolates himself and participates less in family activities. Jason doesn't like to talk about what happened to him, even though he thinks about it every day. Each painful step reminds him of the accident and all the changes that have taken place in his life since then. Now constantly in the grip of severe anxiety, Jason can no longer cope with it alone. He needs to seek specialized help.

CATASTROPHIZING

Catastrophic thinking, or catastrophizing, offers one of the best examples of the impact of thoughts on pain perception. Often seen in people with chronic pain, catastrophizing is fuelled by anything that makes it possible to view an event from a tragic perspective and therefore to fear dreadful consequences. In 1995, Dr. Michael Sullivan and his

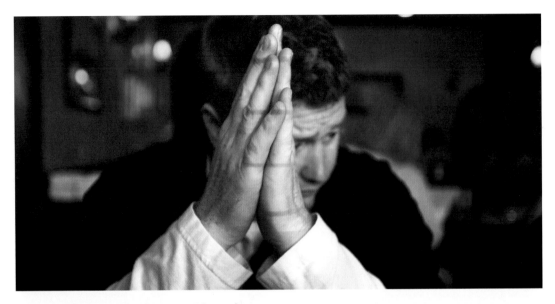

Post-Traumatic Stress Disorder

Post-traumatic stress disorder (PTSD) is a serious form of anxiety observed in some people who have experienced or seen traumatic events involving the threat of death or serious injury (major accidents, assaults, rapes, wars, genocides) and who have reacted with intense fear or feelings of helplessness or horror. These people then experience powerful anxiety accompanied by memories of the event (flashbacks or nightmares) that disrupt everyday activities, avoidance behaviour, and problems managing emotions (introversion, insensitivity), as well as a number of mood disorders (irritability, difficulties concentrating). In some cases, these symptoms are accompanied by physical effects typical of anxiety, such as restlessness, heart palpitations, nausea, and headaches.

The negative memories of the trauma can also make the pain more intense by causing people to withdraw into themselves and display avoidance behaviour. As for the pain, it may be a reminder of the circumstances surrounding the physical trauma, like the loss of a loved one or of one's own physical abilities, such as an amputation, thus creating psychological stress that makes it worse.

colleagues divided this kind of thinking into three distinct yet interrelated parts.

Rumination is the stage where people pay attention only to the pain and can't control their recurring thoughts: "I can't stop thinking about how much it hurts."

Magnification is when people tend to exaggerate the pain's unpleasant effect and anticipate negative consequences: "I'm afraid that something serious is going to happen."

Helplessness is the stage where people really no longer have confidence in personal or medical resources to manage their situation: "There's nothing I can do to reduce my pain."

It's important to recognize a catastrophic thought when it arises, as this factor is, just like depression, closely related to the deterioration in quality of life observed in some people with chronic pain. Studies show that in the case of several types of chronic pain, people who get into the habit of catastrophic thinking say that their pain is more intense, are at greater risk of disability and incapacity in the workplace, and respond less well to medical treatments (Adams et al., 2007).

This negative feedback loop is largely triggered by the fear that is such an integral part of catastrophizing (Figure 27). People who confront pain directly, remain realistic and optimistic about the possibility of finding a solution, follow their therapeutic regimen to the letter, and don't view pain as dangerous, but instead as an ordeal they can overcome, have a high probability of making a better recovery and regaining a good quality of life. Conversely, when pain is interpreted in a catastrophic way, this negative assessment is a precursor to fear-related pain and thus magnifies the pain's intensity. This leads to avoidance and escapist behaviours that reduce the possibility of taking part in any activity whatsoever, and

lead to repercussions very often associated with this kind of avoidance, both emotional (irritability, frustration, depression) and physical (incapacity, disability).

DEPRESSION

People coping with persistent pain often feel they have lost control of their life and are watching it pass slowly by without being able to play an active role in it. The feeling of helplessness is all the more strong when they feel they are alone and abandoned, sometimes even by the medical community, which can't seem to find a cure for their pain. Discouraged by having to fight continually without finding even temporary respite, they feel very sad about what they have become, unable to see the light at the end of the tunnel and draw on their own resources to manage the pain that has taken over their life (Figure 28). These moments of depression may be short-lived: since chronic pain is an exhausting experience, both psychologically and physically, it's normal to feel down from time to time. However, when they occur over long periods of time, these moments of sadness can

THE FEAR-AVOIDANCE MODEL

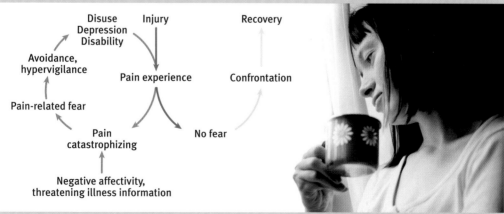

FIGURE 27

Vlaeyen and Linton, 2000

THE THREE COMPONENTS
OF DEPRESSION

Affective

- Loss of interest, enjoyment
- Sadness
- Depression
- Despair
- Powerlessness

Behavioural

- Loss of motivation
- Loss of or increase in appetite
- Hypersomnia/insomnia
- Restlessness
- Weeping
- Fatigue
- Weight gain or loss

Cognitive (thinking)

- Concentration or attention problems
- Discouragement
- Feeling of failure
- Guilt
- Disappointment
- Suicidal thoughts
- Indecision
- Declining self-esteem

FIGURE 28

cause great distress and turn into episodes of depression that are sometimes serious.

Just like other psychological disorders, depression remains an illness poorly understood by the general public, with many viewing it as a minor mood disorder that people can overcome simply "by thinking about something else." In fact, depression is a serious neurophysiological disorder, caused by imbalances in the levels of certain neurotransmitters involved in emotional well-being, and it must be diagnosed as quickly as possible to prevent it from getting worse.

Depression is often associated with chronic pain: people coping with persistent pain are twice as likely to be depressed as the general population. Approximately 32 percent of women and 22 percent of men with chronic pain show symptoms of depression; the seriousness of these symptoms depends on several factors, including the type of pain, its intensity, its duration, the availability of the sufferer's personal resources, and other factors in their lives before, during and after the onset of the pain (Statistics Canada, 2000–2001). Sometimes depression also triggers pain, as if the body were physically expressing its inner misery, but in most cases it's a consequence of chronic pain.

There is an overall loss of "life force," meaning that people lose their confidence and self-esteem, feel a great weariness with respect to all the events happening in their daily life, dwell on past events and can't help having a pessimistic view of their current and future existence.

For chronic pain sufferers, depression has serious repercussions for physical and psychological health. Depression negatively influences pain perception by disrupting the descending pathways controlled by the brain. People who are depressed also respond less well to suggested treatments (physical, medical, and pharmacological) because they have difficulty getting motivated, "taking charge of themselves," and fully understanding the concrete actions they have to take to manage their pain properly. At the same time, depression heightens the feeling of helplessness and despair they feel about their pain, and patients frequently develop very poor self-esteem, seeing themselves only from the perspective of pain, dependence, and disability. In the most serious cases, a depression like this triggers dark thoughts: patients may consider suicide to end the misery and a life that no longer has meaning (see "When Pain Triggers Suicidal Thoughts," below).

Catastrophizing and depression are two striking examples of the huge influence thoughts and emotions have on adaptation to chronic pain. By profoundly disrupting normal emotional processes, these two pathological states cause a number of changes in attitudes, thinking, and even certain physiological systems that, tog-ether, negatively influence the pain experience, both from the point of view of its intensity (increased inflammation, hypersensitivity) and its impacts on people's lives (physical disability) (Figure 29).

To adapt to chronic pain, all the mechanisms, strategies, and tools that can help people modify their emotions, thoughts, and harmful behaviours must be called on. There's no universal prescription for effectively managing the impact of chronic pain on the life of a particular person, but studies conducted in recent decades by a number of doctors, psychologists, and other health professionals have made it possible to identify a certain number of parameters that can help mitigate it significantly. To learn to live better with chronic pain, we have to broaden our horizons and consider the entire body of knowledge acquired in recent years as to the best ways to fight this illness. Let's begin with the absolutely essential role played by pain medications.

When Pain Triggers Suicidal Thoughts

Helen, aged seventy, is exhausted from living with a pain in the shoulder that has been gnawing at her since she fell down the stairs nearly twenty years ago and has become more difficult to manage in the past three years without her knowing why. She feels she has no energy left to carry on and would like to end her life, as she believes it no longer has any meaning. Not only is she sad, but she's seeing her autonomy diminish and needs help from her loved ones to carry out certain activities. Discouraged and ashamed, Helen doesn't know how to cope with this hurdle, despite having overcome so many in her lifetime. When she goes to bed, she hopes she won't wake up the next morning.

Many people with chronic pain have at one time or another thought about taking their own life. For most of them, these thoughts are passive, that is, there is no concrete plan to carry them out. These people don't really want to die — what they want is not to suffer anymore. These thoughts attest to the unbearable pain they live with day after day. Most of these people see suicide more as a solution for their general unhappiness than just for their pain; they have reached the limits of their resources, feel excluded from society and their families, and can no longer find valid reasons to stay alive. They've simply had it.

Yet, as we will see in Chapter 6, several solutions for alleviating pain do exist.

THE INFLUENCE OF DEPRESSION AND CATASTROPHIZING ON CHRONIC PAIN

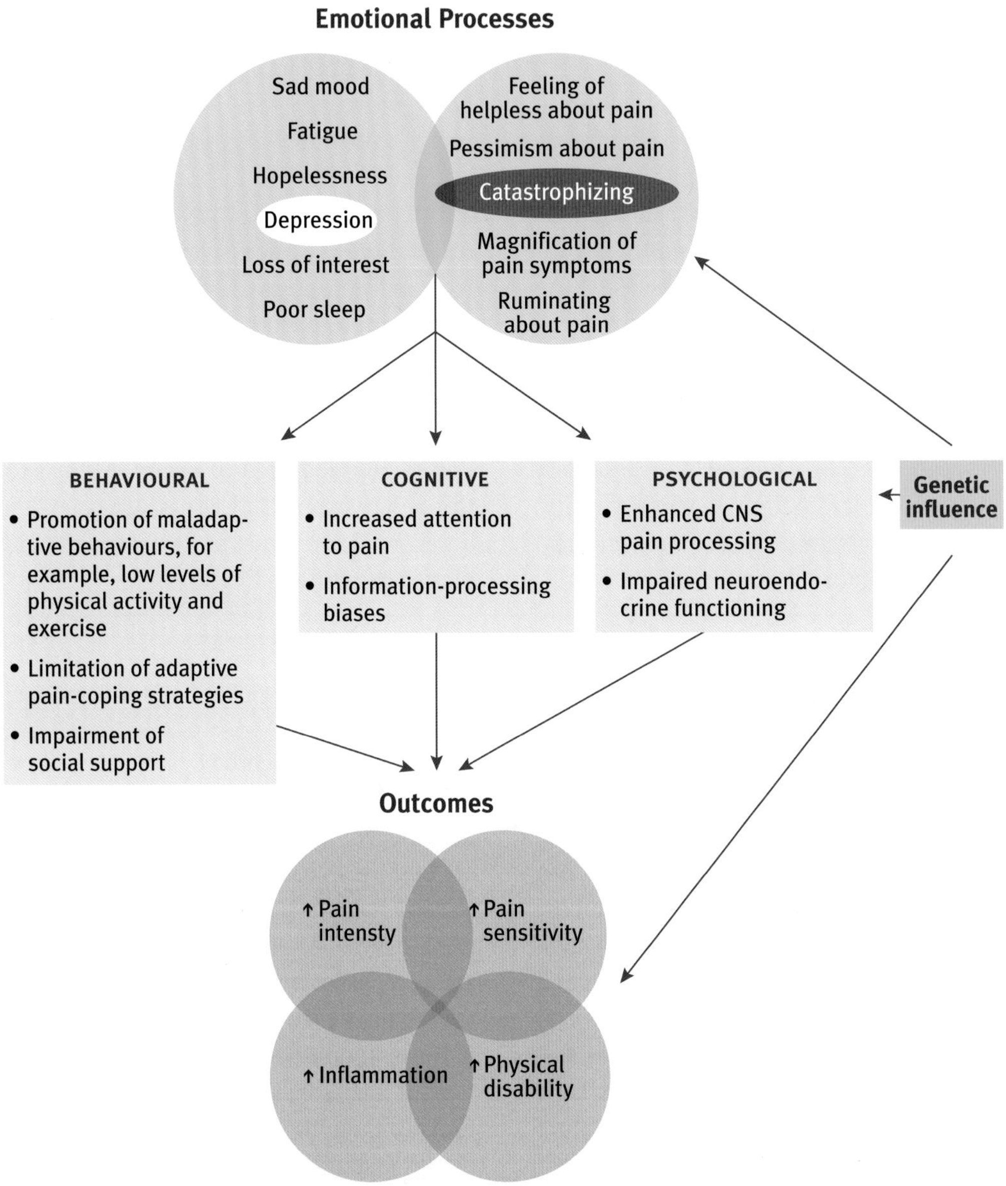

Emotional Processes

Sad mood

Fatigue

Hopelessness

Depression

Loss of interest

Poor sleep

Feeling of helpless about pain

Pessimism about pain

Catastrophizing

Magnification of pain symptoms

Ruminating about pain

BEHAVIOURAL

- Promotion of maladaptive behaviours, for example, low levels of physical activity and exercise
- Limitation of adaptive pain-coping strategies
- Impairment of social support

COGNITIVE

- Increased attention to pain
- Information-processing biases

PSYCHOLOGICAL

- Enhanced CNS pain processing
- Impaired neuroendocrine functioning

Genetic influence

Outcomes

↑ Pain intensty

↑ Pain sensitivity

↑ Inflammation

↑ Physical disability

FIGURE 1

Adapted from Edwards et. al., 2011

In Summary

- The emotions experienced—anger, guilt, shame and fear—have a particularly strong impact on the quality of life of people with chronic pain.

- Chronic pain causes changes in thinking and behaviour, which in turn can greatly increase the intensity and perception of pain.

- Various forms of anxiety and depression are the psychological consequences of chronic pain most often diagnosed in sufferers.

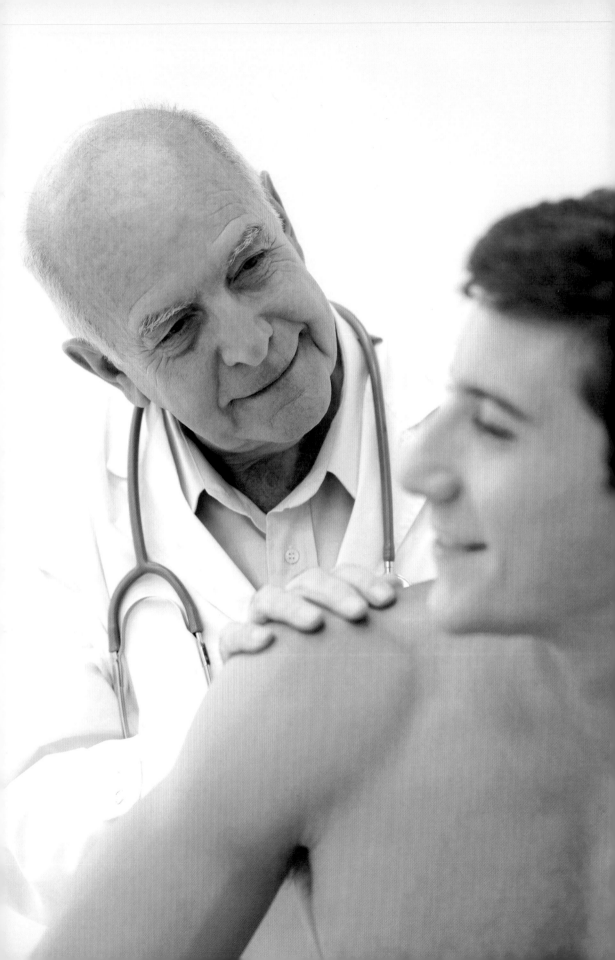

CHAPTER 5

The Therapeutic Challenge: About Medical Treatments*

Cure sometimes, relieve often, and comfort always.
— MEDICAL ADAGE ATTRIBUTED
TO AMBROISE PARÉ, SIXTEENTH CENTURY

In the perpetual search for ways to cure or, at the very least, relieve pain, human beings have identified a wide array of plants with therapeutic properties (see p. 112). This pain-relieving and plant-sourced "medicine chest" has played a major role in enhancing the quality of life of countless people and still has a large influence on the medical approach to pain. Indeed, regardless of whether they are salicylates like aspirin or opiates derived from morphine, most current pain control molecules are produced in one way or another from plants with analgesic properties identified several thousand years ago.

COMPLEX AND SUBOPTIMAL TREATMENT

To men and women in modern industrialized societies, having to "tolerate" pain may seem incomprehensible. Today we enjoy exceptional living conditions and unprecedented comfort, unimaginable just a few decades ago. The excellence of modern medicine, capable of relieving and curing an ever-growing number of ills, also contributes to this quality of life: while pain remains an unavoidable reality of life, usually viewed with anxiety, we have access to a wide range of medical options to prevent it or at least minimize its harmful impact on our lives. Except when it indicates an injury or an acute illness (appendicitis, heart attack), pain is never a positive sign; it's a negative and anxiety-provoking experience that we try to fight using all the medical and technological means at our disposal.

Yet, the prevalence of chronic pain in modern society reminds us that the battle is far from won and that, on the contrary, it faces challenging obstacles. On the one hand, pain is an extremely complex

* Chapter written with the collaboration of Dr. David Lussier.

physiological process, whose treatment may produce highly variable results. On the other, it's a subjective sensation that differs considerably from person to person; this complicates the task of the medical profession in determining the kind and dosage of medications best adapted to relieve patients' pain, without at the same time causing serious side effects. Despite considerable medical progress in recent years, pain is still too often treated in a suboptimal way, causing unjustified physical and psychological stress in a sizable number of patients. At its meeting in Montreal in 2010, this concern led the International Association for the Study of Pain (IASP), an association with 7,500 members in 129 countries around the world, to publish a declaration reaffirming that adequate pain management is a fundamental right of human beings, and that as a result it must become an absolute priority for medical treatment. Some progress on this front has indeed been made. For example, initiatives have been put forward to better train health professionals in how to treat pain; these initiatives have produced very encouraging results with a direct impact on the care all of these professionals provide to patients.

PAIN TREATMENT

Although treating chronic pain appropriately is difficult, the medical profession is not totally lacking in resources for dealing with this illness. In many cases, it's possible to reduce the intensity of the pain substantially using medications, invasive procedures like injections, implants, or even specific surgical procedures, and

these methods are an essential part of any pain management strategy. Medical intervention also plays a predominant role in relieving a number of the after-effects of pain (sleep disturbances, lack of appetite, depression) and thus gives patients the respite they need to acquire the skills essential for managing it.

The ultimate goal of proper chronic pain treatment is to improve the quality of life of people in pain. For this to happen, the pain must be assessed as accurately as possible and the pharmacological, medical, physical, and psychological treatments most likely to improve the patient's condition must be identified.

PAIN ASSESSMENT

To fully identify needs for medication, invasive interventions and non-drug treatments, the pain and its various components must be properly assessed. A number of very detailed pieces of information are required to enable medical professionals — doctors, nurses, psychologists, physiotherapists, occupational therapists, or others — to take the most effective action.

Assessing the Person

Needless to say, you can't assess someone's pain without looking at the whole person; by definition, each kind of pain is unique because it's perceived differently by each sufferer. People who live with it daily are the best placed to describe what they are feeling and the pain they describe must be the starting point in the assessment process.

"Talking about" their pain, and describing its physical and emotional effects, is a difficult task for patients, who are often not

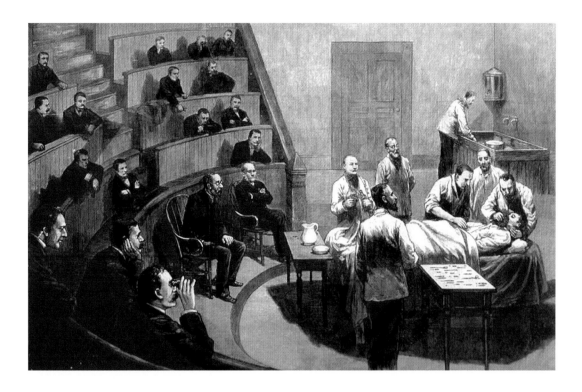

Painless Operations

For much of our past, except for the occasional use of certain plants such as mandragore, operations, whether they were to amputate a limb, remove a cancerous tumour, or simply treat a toothache, were performed "cold," without any anesthetic. History is full of ghastly tales of people who endured these kinds of surgery while being held down by the strength of several men and screaming throughout the entire operation. For doctors, who had the thankless job of curing patients while making them suffer, this pain was an unavoid-able consequence if they hoped to save the patient. This resignation to pain was largely due to the lack of genuine anesthetics: opium was risky, since in high doses it can cause death; alcohol was too unpredictable because of its impact on the patient's personality; cold was not very useful for more invasive surgery. It was not until the beginning of the nineteenth century that a growing concern for patients' welfare acted as a catalyst in identifying new anesthetics, a quest that would eventually lead to the use of ether, beginning in 1846.

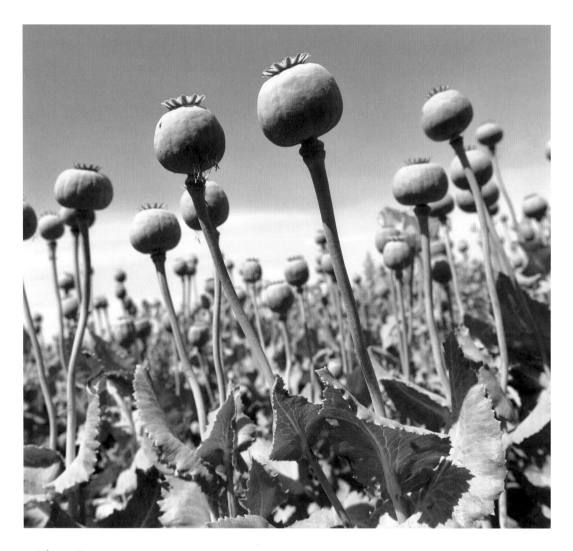

Plant Doctors

Among the many medicinal plants discovered over the centuries, three have especially interesting analgesic properties.

OPIUM

The opium poppy (Papaver somniferum) was already being cultivated in Europe at least seven thousand years ago, likely for the protein and oil in its seeds. But there is no doubt that its analgesic properties were soon noticed, especially by the ancient Greeks, who described the analgesic effect of what they called opios, the sap harvested from the poppy's flower. This sap contains about forty alkaloids, the most abundant being morphine (10–15 percent), papaverine (4–5 percent), and codeine (1–3 percent).

These molecules play a key role in defending the plant from predators. Poppy alkaloids are the plant-based molecules with the strongest analgesic action; their effect stems from their ability to mimic the analgesic action of endorphins in the central nervous system. Opium's powerful analgesic effect has led to its use in relieving a whole range of ailments, from simple discomfort to the most serious injuries. The main component of opium, morphine, is still an essential element in care given to patients with severe pain.

WILLOW

Willow is one of the oldest remedies used to soothe pain and fevers. Already mentioned in Mesopotamia at least seven thousand years ago, as well as in the oldest Egyptian medical treatises, the bark of the white willow (Salix alba) was held in high esteem by Hippocrates (460–377 BCE), who recommended it for relieving the pain of childbirth, among other things. North American Indians also used decoctions made from the bark and roots of the pussy willow (Salix discolor) as a multipurpose analgesic remedy.

In 1897 German chemist Felix Hoffmann, working for the Bayer company, succeeded in synthesizing acetylsalicylic acid — the aspirin that has since become so much a part of our daily lives — from the active ingredient in willow bark, salacin. The first therapeutic molecule created in a laboratory, aspirin has played a key role in the development of the pharmaceutical industry and is, without doubt, history's most successful drug. Nearly three thousand aspirin tablets are still produced and consumed every second worldwide, for a total of eighty billion per year!

CANNABIS

Likely native to Central Asia, Cannabis sativa is a woody plant that has been used for several millennia as a source of fibres for making rope and cloth. It's thought that it was the Chinese, around two thousand years BCE, who were the first to use cannabis to treat various kinds of pain. In addition, the plant's hallucinogenic properties did not go unnoticed, and most of the peoples of antiquity associated the mental euphoria induced by cannabis with magical, mystical, or social experiences. Today, cannabis remains inseparable from cultural traditions in certain parts of the world, notably India and Jamaica, and it's by far the most common recreational drug on the planet, with nearly 200 million regular users.

It was only in 1964 that Raphael Mechoulam isolated the active ingredient in cannabis, the Δ9-tetrahydrocannabinol, commonly known as THC. The analgesic effect of THC comes from its interaction with certain receptors that reduce the transmission of painful nerve impulses to the spinal cord and brain stem.

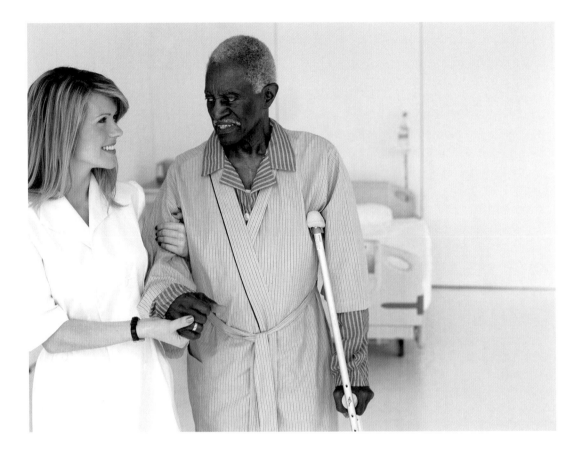

very inclined to discuss the misery they experience daily, since discussing it plunges them back into a world they are trying to escape. It's therefore important to give people time and gentle support to encourage them to express as freely as possible the thoughts and emotions they experience on a daily basis.

Aspects to be Assessed

The pain's location. The first step is to accurately determine where the pain is. Where is it actually located, where does it start from, and where does it go to? A person may for example have lower back pain that remains localized or radiates down one leg or even both; depending on the situation, the diagnosis can be different,

and so can suggested treatments. If there is more than one painful spot, the pain can also be "mapped" — sketched on an image of the human body to create an exact overall picture.

The Pain's intensity. To treat pain effectively, it's absolutely necessary to know how intense it is. Since no machine can measure pain, a numerical scale from 0 to 10, on which 0 means no pain and 10, the worst pain imaginable, is generally used. A measurement of this kind is of course imprecise but it nonetheless makes it possible to obtain indispensable information about the intensity of the pain experienced by the patient at the time or in the recent past.

Factors influencing the pain's intensity. Intensity can vary considerably depending on time of day, the kind of activities undertaken, temperature, stress level, etc. This information is important in determining the treatment conditions most likely to alleviate the pain.

The disruptive nature of the pain. The emotional aspect of pain is measured using a numerical scale similar to the one used to measure its intensity. The sufferer is asked, "To what extent, on a scale of 0 to 10, does your pain bother you?" Responses can vary greatly, independent of the intensity of the pain that is physically felt. For example, a person might rate the intensity of his or her pain at 7 out of 10, but the level of disruption at 5 out of 10, or conversely, the pain might have an intensity level of 4 out of 10 and a level of disruption of 8 out of 10.

The description of the pain. The words used by patients to describe pain are very important. Professor Ronald Melzack has developed a questionnaire — the McGill Pain Questionnaire — that lists a series of words and adjectives describing pain. These assist in making a diagnosis since pain that tingles or causes numbness is different from dull or throbbing pain (Figure 30).

Assessing the consequences of pain and emotions in daily life.

- The person's level of functioning. An attempt will be made to determine how the pain interferes with everyday activities — work, household chores, leisure activities. As we saw in Chapter 3, pain has an impact on every aspect of sufferers' lives and these impacts must be assessed.
- The emotional state. What emotions is the person experiencing? How is the person feeling? What are the

circumstances that caused the pain? What was the stress level before and after the triggering event?
- The quality of sleep, nutrition, and physical exercise. These aspects have to be considered because they are affected by pain, influence its perception, and can even modify the effect of treatments.

Assessing expectations. What is the person hoping for? Relief or to be pain free? An improvement in quality of life, in their ability to function, in their general health? Less psychological distress? These expectations must be clarified during the assessment, as they will serve as benchmarks when establishing a treatment plan.

Several other physical and radiological examinations may be necessary to determine the kind of pain in question, as well as the underlying mechanisms that are likely at play. It is then up to doctors to use the results of these more precise tests to diagnose what is causing the pain.

———

These are only a few of the aspects assessed during a first meeting with a doctor, and the actual medical examination is more thorough than this short description indicates. The same is true of the assessments made by other health professionals, who will ask questions more specifically related to their fields of expertise, underlining the importance of a good working relationship between patients and these professionals. In addition, there are a number of questionnaires that help provide a more complete picture of each of the elements listed here. In short, ever

THE MCGILL PAIN QUESTIONNAIRE: WORDS DESCRIBING PAIN

These groups of words are used to describe every kind of pain. Some of these words may correspond to the pain you are feeling right now. Please check those (one per group) that best describe your pain. Leave out any group that does not contain a word describing your pain.

1. ☐ Flickering
   ☐ Quivering
   ☐ Pulsing
   ☐ Throbbing
   ☐ Beating
   ☐ Pounding

2. ☐ Jumping
   ☐ Flashing
   ☐ Shooting

3. ☐ Pricking
   ☐ Boring
   ☐ Drilling
   ☐ Stabbing

4. ☐ Sharp
   ☐ Cutting
   ☐ Lacerating

5. ☐ Pinching
   ☐ Pressing
   ☐ Gnawing
   ☐ Cramping
   ☐ Crushing

6. ☐ Tugging
   ☐ Pulling
   ☐ Wrenching

7. ☐ Hot
   ☐ Burning
   ☐ Scalding
   ☐ Searing

8. ☐ Tingling
   ☐ Itchy
   ☐ Smarting
   ☐ Stinging

9. ☐ Dull
   ☐ Sore
   ☐ Hurting
   ☐ Aching
   ☐ Heavy

10. ☐ Tender
    ☐ Taut (tight)
    ☐ Rasping
    ☐ Splitting

11. ☐ Tiring
    ☐ Exhausting

12. ☐ Sickening
    ☐ Suffocating

13. ☐ Fearful
    ☐ Frightful
    ☐ Terrifying

14. ☐ Punishing
    ☐ Grueling
    ☐ Cruel
    ☐ Vicious
    ☐ Killing

15. ☐ Wretching
    ☐ Blinding

16. ☐ Annoying
    ☐ Troublesome
    ☐ Miserable
    ☐ Intense
    ☐ Unbearable

17. ☐ Spreading
    ☐ Radiating
    ☐ Penetrating
    ☐ Piercing

18. ☐ Tight
    ☐ Numb
    ☐ Drawing
    ☐ Squeezing
    ☐ Tearing

19. ☐ Cool
    ☐ Cold
    ☐ Freezing

20. ☐ Nagging
    ☐ Nauseating
    ☐ Agonizing
    ☐ Dreadful
    ☐ Torturing

FIGURE 30

Adapted from Melzack, 1975

more precise assessment tools assist clinicians in all specialties to form an accurate overall picture of the pain and those living with it.

MEDICATIONS

Obviously, we can't talk about relieving pain without talking about medications. The vast majority of chronic pain sufferers take medication from one or several classes of analgesic drugs daily, which help, at least in part, to alleviate their pain (Figure 31).

All of these medications act on one or the other of the pathways that transmit or integrate the pain signal, either in the peripheral or central nervous system (Figure 32). For example, non-opiate analgesics like acetaminophen or aspirin interfere in the production of inflammatory molecules at the source, thus reducing the pain signal before it reaches the spinal cord and the brain. Opiates, on the other hand, act mainly on the central nervous system and prevent the pain signal coming from the periphery from reaching the various regions of the brain dealing with pain perception. By means of these drugs, as well as several other molecules with analgesic properties, the pain sensation can be considerably reduced; they are thus indispensable therapeutic tools for treating chronic pain.

The principles governing the therapeutic use of analgesics are complex and their description is beyond the scope of this book. We should mention, however, that a doctor's choice of a medication is influenced by five main factors.

The Kind of Pain

Each medication has a different window of effectiveness, depending on the mechanisms causing the pain sensation. For example, medications for neuropathic pain are different from those used to relieve muscle pain. In some cases, a combination of different drugs is a better option, since a drug that hasn't been very effective in relieving pain may prove more useful when combined with another drug.

Pain Intensity

Moderate pain will not be treated in the same way as pain identified as severe. Some practice guidelines have been developed based on pain intensity to make it easier to determine the choice of treatment; their validity has been questioned however, at least in part, because the intensity of the pain must not be the only determining factor in treatment choice.

Individual Differences

People respond differently to the same medication, even when the kind of pain being treated is similar. Their age must also be considered, with the elderly often having a response and tolerance to drugs very different from that of younger people. A patient's medical history, current state of health, previous problems with

THE MAIN TYPES OF MEDICATION USED TO TREAT CHRONIC PAIN IN EUROPE

Types of drugs used

Anti-inflammatories (non-steroidal) **44%**

Weak opiates **23%**

Acetaminophen (paracetamol) **18%**

Strong opiates **5%**

FIGURE 31   Adapted from Breivik et all., 2006

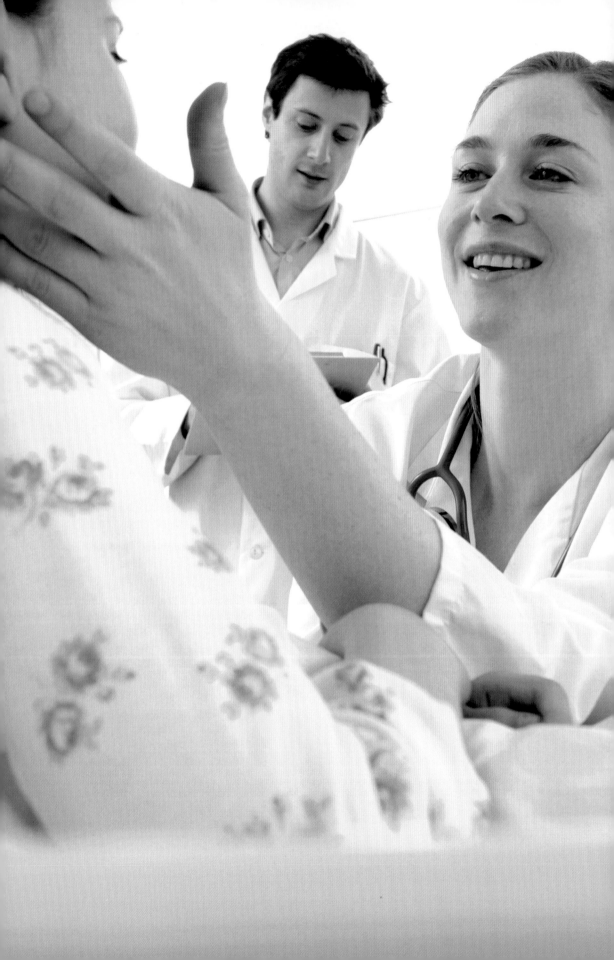

substance dependence or abuse and psychological condition are also aspects to assess in selecting drugs.

Side Effects

All medications have undesirable and unpredictable side effects, whose seriousness varies considerably from person to person. These side effects are often a major obstacle in treating chronic pain, making it necessary to avoid administering certain very effective medications or sufficiently high doses to produce a therapeutic effect.

Patient-Doctor Collaboration

Choosing a medication requires close monitoring of both the progression of the pain and the positive or negative effects of the treatment being tested. This is the job of the attending physician, the only one who has a global knowledge of the patient's file and who can modify the pharmacological approach to achieve the greatest possible pain relief.

But while the responsibility for identifying the best pain-relieving medication falls on the doctor, patients also have to participate actively in the process, notably by following the treatment to the letter (adherence) and being aware of the treatment's limits and possible side effects (Figure 33). To do this, they must keep a record of the medication's effects.

MANAGING UNPLEASANT OR HARMFUL SIDE EFFECTS

It's very important to learn to manage the side effects associated with most medications. Initially, patience is required: when a medication is first prescribed or its dose is increased, the length of time

the body needs to adapt to it varies, and any unpleasant side effects may disappear quite quickly. The pros and cons of a medication must also be assessed: do its benefits in improving quality of life outweigh its unpleasant effects? The delicate balance between the therapeutic effect of a drug and its undesirable side effects can change over time, and these components must therefore be regularly reassessed. However, if a drug's undesirable effects last longer than a few days or become very severe, the doctor who prescribed it must be consulted urgently to discuss the problem and change the approach. Managing the side effects of medications is as important as managing the positive effects of pain relief.

COMPLIANCE TO TREATMENT

Despite their key role in managing their own pain, many patients remain extremely wary about the usefulness of medications, in spite of the physical pain and suffering they have to tolerate (Figure 34). Sometimes, people even prefer not to take a drug or only take their medications irregularly, often as a last resort when the pain becomes too severe. Fear of losing self-control, of not knowing who they are anymore, mistrust about the long-term effects of drugs on the organism, or the risk of dependence are the main reasons given to justify this behaviour (Figure 35). This is especially common in those who have seen loved ones react negatively to certain drugs, experience side effects or major complications, and lose their ability to function.

Dependence is a genuine risk with some classes of drugs (notably the opioids), especially when they are not

THE MAIN MEDICATIONS USED TO TREAT NON-CANCEROUS CHRONIC PAIN

Classes of medication	Characteristics
NON-OPIAT ANALGESICS • ASS (asprin) • Acetaminophen • NSAIDs (non-steroidal anti-inflammatories)	• Are the best-known and most-used drugs in the world. • Have analgesic properties. • Some have a direct effect on the injury.
COANALGESICS (EXAMPLES) • Antidepressants • Anticonvulsants	• Medications developed for problems other than pain but which have an analgesic effect. • The choice is made based on several pain assessment criteria. • Some antidepressants target very specific types of pain (e.g. neuropathic pain, fibromyalgia, or osteoarthritis). When they are prescribed to treat pain, this has nothing at all to do with their effect on depression. They are effective even if the patient isn't depressed and are usually prescribed in weaker doses than for depression. • Antidepressants may also be prescribed to treat depression in someone who is both in pain and depressed; this may have a positive impact on both conditions. • Anticonvulsants are normally prescribed for neuropathic pain and fibromyalgia. Their effect on pain is completely independent of their effect on epilepsy. Like epilepsy, pain is sometimes caused by increased activity in nerve cells. By reducing this activity, anticonvulsants can decrease pain.

FIGURE 32

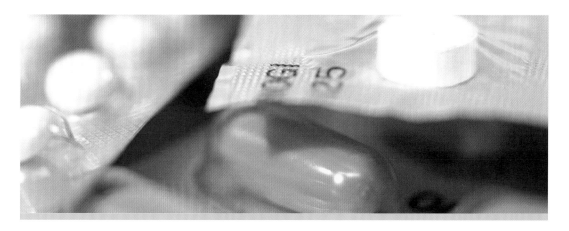

Classes of medication	Characteristics
OPIODS (EXAMPLES) • Codeine • Oxycodone • Morphine (natural opiate) • Hydromorphone • Fentanyl • Methadone • Tramadol • Tapentadol	• Have analgesic properties • Can be administered by mouth (per os), rectally, subcutaneously, intramuscularly, or intravenously, depending on the desired speed and duration of the drug's action. • Are produced in both immediate-release and extended-release forms (fast-acting and slow-acting). • Act on the central nervous system and (or) have an analgesic effect right at the source of the pain.
CANNABINOIDS	• Like opioids, cannabinoids occur naturally in the human body (endogenous cannabinoids). In patients with chronic pain, synthetic cannabinoids may be prescribed in drug form to relieve pain. • In addition to cannabinoids given in the form of medication (pills, sprays), inhaled cannabis may be administered to treat pain. Several studies are underway on people to definitively confirm their true analgesic potential, already observed in cells and animals, as well as in some people who use them.

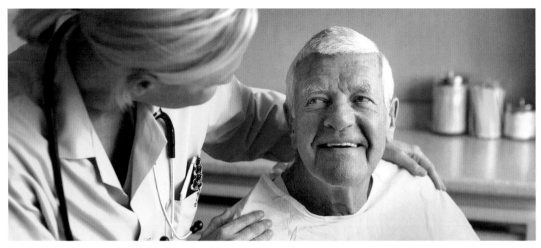

MEDICATION: WHO DOES WHAT?

Medical staff's responsibilities	Your responsibilities as a patient
Properly assesses the pain situation and its impacts on the patient's life.	Provide all necessary details to facilitate this assessment.
Presents the treatments and the reasons for suggesting them.	Make sure to understand fully the reasons for taking a medication.
Clearly explains how to take the medication and for how long.	Take the medication according to the prescription: don't self-medicate.
Discusses possible disagreeable side effects.	Take note of all the effects, both positive and negative, associated with taking the medication.
Makes sure the patient won't run out of pills before the next appointment.	Make sure the renewal will be done before the pills run out, don't wait until the last minute, manage your pills carefully.
Knows about all the medications the patient is taking.	Keep an up-to-date list at hand of medications being taken and provide it as needed.
Takes the time necessary to really listen.	Express yourself clearly, make a note of thoughts to discuss, prepare for your appointment with the doctor.
	Don't consult several doctors at the same time for the same problem, and don't "go shopping" for doctors. When you're in a therapeutic relationship with a doctor, the treatment will be much more effective and safe if one doctor alone prescribes pain-control medications.

FIGURE 33

taken as prescribed. This can cause confusion, for some people, about the terms used when referring to medications, like dependence, tolerance and addiction. These distinct terms must not be confused, as the problems they refer to are not the same (Figure 36).

A medication that's correctly prescribed, taken as directed, with a specific therapeutic goal and under medical supervision can not only relieve pain but also promote a better quality of life. Of course, if a drug is unnecessary, taking it is useless; however, when it means a significantly better quality of life, it's important to conquer the fear we might have about it and take it responsibly.

People treated with drugs do not lose control of themselves; quite the opposite — by choosing rationally to use all available resources to improve their condition, they exercise more control over their lives and enhance their chances of rehabilitation. If you have a chronic illness that could benefit from the positive impact of certain medications, why not consider them? You never know what treatment the pain might respond to, which is why it's important to keep an open mind about the therapeutic potential of the medication your doctor suggests.

This open-minded attitude is important, because identifying the most appropriate medications for relieving pain can sometimes turn out to be a long and arduous process involving much trial and error. While most of the time a drug's therapeutic effect is already known or predictable, the doctor cannot know in advance what its impact will be on particular patients, nor how they will react to treatment. The dose administered, the time

PRESCRIPTION MEDICATION USE IN PEOPLE WITH CHRONIC PAIN

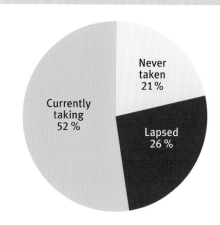

Never taken 21%

Currently taking 52%

Lapsed 26%

REASON WHY LAPSED

Lack of need   64%

Manage/live with pain   19%

Pain not bad enough   15%

Pain gone/no longer have pain/pain under control   14%

Not needed/no longer necessary   11%

Side effects/other negative impacts   34%

Too many side effects/do not like side effects   14%

Do not want to take any more pain medicine   11%

Medication ineffective   9%

Taking too much medication   3%

Can be addictive   2%

Using alternative treatments   7%

Health/medical reasons   7%

Prefer non-prescription medicine/doctor recommended non-prescription medicine   5%

Have not been to/seen doctor   2%

FIGURE 34   Breivik et al., 2006

of day when the drug is taken and the occurrence and seriousness of side effects are all unpredictable variables that differ considerably from one person to another and complicate pain management. Although this is a frustrating stage, it's essential not to get discouraged if the therapeutic effect is not adequate or side effects occur.

On the contrary, you have to become even more careful about your medication and avoid taking a drug without knowing why. You need to be sure you know the name of the medication, how long it will be used, and why the doctor has prescribed it, and keep detailed notes about its negative effects. With this information, the usefulness and suitability of all medications being taken can be ensured and it becomes easier to monitor their effectiveness. Also, and most importantly, it means you maintain control both over yourself and the drugs you are taking. You should not stop taking a drug without being supervised by the doctor who prescribed it or the doctor who is monitoring it, nor, especially, should you "go shopping" — seeing several doctors to obtain other painkillers. This can have undesirable effects on the treatment (drug interactions, risk of dependence) and break the bond of trust between patient and doctor. These steps are important, for when the medication is appropriate, taken correctly and re-evaluated regularly to ensure its

STATED ATTITUDES AND BELIEFS ABOUT PAIN TREATMENTS

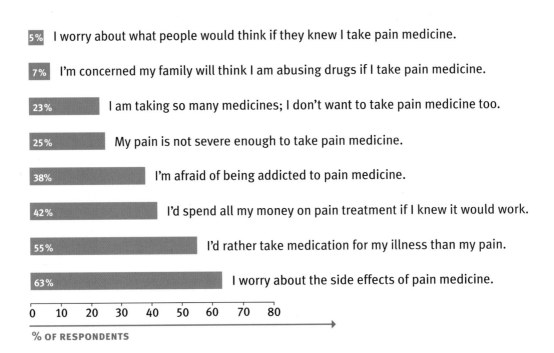

5% I worry about what people would think if they knew I take pain medicine.

7% I'm concerned my family will think I am abusing drugs if I take pain medicine.

23% I am taking so many medicines; I don't want to take pain medicine too.

25% My pain is not severe enough to take pain medicine.

38% I'm afraid of being addicted to pain medicine.

42% I'd spend all my money on pain treatment if I knew it would work.

55% I'd rather take medication for my illness than my pain.

63% I worry about the side effects of pain medicine.

% OF RESPONDENTS

FIGURE 35   Breivik et al., 2006

effectiveness, it can be an indispensable help to sufferers, setting them free from the constant pressure of pain, so that they can devote their physical and psychological energy to more constructive activities that enhance their quality of life.

MEDICAL INTERVENTIONS

In order to treat pain properly, several kinds of treatment must be considered. In combination with drugs, the doctor may suggest other interventions that work in various ways and provide additional relief.

INJECTIONS

Injections are given in a specific part of the body, in the spot where the pain is felt or close to it, and the type of medication injected varies depending on the desired results and the kind of pain. Injections are most common in the joints, muscles or close to nerves. The usual injection sites are trigger points located in muscles that are sensitive to touch, joints where there is inflammation and pain, or the spinal column — like the epidural, which can be given in the cervical, dorsal, or lumbar region. The choice of these interventions is based on the same criteria as for medications and requires a discussion with the doctor to determine the one best suited to a patient's needs.

NERVE STIMULATION

Pain relief can sometimes be achieved by stimulating the nerves that transmit pain. The main techniques used are TENS(Transcutaneous Electrical Nerve Stimulation) and neurostimulation.

During TENS, electrodes are placed on the affected area to maximize pain relief (for example, on the lower back for lumbar pain). These electrodes send electrical impulses that stimulate nerves according to a pre-determined frequency, intensity, and duration. The pain relief can be considerable for many people and can be even more effective when TENS is combined with other methods.

In neurostimulation, electrodes are implanted in the body, right at the source of the pain. The nerves are then stimulated, much as they are using TENS. This technique's desired objective is to "reprogram" the pain signal generated by the nerve fibres so as to replace the pain sensation with a more pleasant or, at least, less painful one.

There are many other techniques for relieving pain and increasing people's ability to function, one being a morphine pump implant. This field is booming and this kind of treatment can in many cases provide significant relief to patients. These pumps are normally reserved, however, for pain that's resistant to other kinds of treatment.

Non-drug physical techniques, such as applying heat and cold to joints and muscles, can also relieve pain. According to the Ordre professionnel de la physiothérapie du Québec, Quebec's professional physiotherapists' association, applying ice reduces the pain of inflammation, while relaxing the muscles. When the inflammation has died down, heat can also provide pain relief and muscle relaxation. As there are a number of restrictions, it's best to seek advice from a specialist in this field. Lastly, we should remember that physical exercise remains

DEPENDENCE, TOLERANCE, DRUG ADDICTION ...

Physical dependence

State of adaptation in which withdrawal occurs when opioids are suddenly stopped. Seen in most people who take opioids in large doses, uninterrupted, and over a long period. To avoid withdrawal symptoms, it's important not to stop taking opioids suddenly, but instead to do so gradually, following the doctor's instructions.

Not a sign of drug addiction or psychological dependence.

Tolerance

State of adaptation in which higher doses of the same medication are needed to obtain the same analgesic effect. In practice, this happens rarely, and often following prolonged use of high doses of opioids.

It's also possible to develop a tolerance to unpleasant side effects.

Not a sign of drug addiction.

Addiction (toxicomania or psychological dependence)

Illness with genetic, psychosocial, and environmental components. Typically involves a loss of control over the use of drugs, compulsive use, ongoing use despite the consequences, and acute withdrawal symptoms.

When an opioid is prescribed to someone in pain, it's very rare for the patient to develop psychological dependence and not be able to do without it for reasons other than pain, unless drug or alcohol abuse is already a problem.

Pseudotoxicomania (pseudoaddiction)

Being obsessed and focussing all one's energy on obtaining a given drug with the goal of relieving pain.

FIGURE 36

an essential part of pain relief. It prevents the body from getting out of shape by helping lubricate the joints and maintaining a healthy weight.

PAIN MANAGEMENT: A TEAM ACTIVITY

This brief overview of currently available medical approaches for treating chronic pain shows how complex this illness is and underscores the limitations of existing treatments. This is an unusual situation in that, as individuals, we have developed a kind of hands-off, self-effacing approach to how our illnesses are treated, pinning all our hopes on the ability of the medical profession to diag-nose the exact source of the ailment and tackle the problem quickly with drugs or appropriate treatments. In a way, this attitude leads people with chronic pain to put their fates in the hands of medicine, taking for granted that they have no role to play in what happens next, except to take the medications or accept the series of treatments prescribed. This unintentional disengagement from the management of their own illnesses can become a serious handicap in the case of diseases like chronic pain, which require a multidisciplinary approach to treatment.

As we have said several times throughout this book, pain is a complex phenomenon involving not only physical sensations transmitted by nerve fibres, but also the brain's interpretation of these sensations. From a therapeutic point of view, this concept is extremely important, because it implies that chronic pain treatment must target both the physiological and psychological aspects of the pain sensation. In practice,

Charles, 34

Referred to the pain clinic, Charles came for interdisciplinary treatment for neck pain that had tormented him since he was body-checked during a friendly hockey game a few years ago. He said he was very hesitant about taking any kind of medication. He had seen his mother die of cancer five years earlier and witnessed the impact that certain drugs had had on her. When the team suggested a drug treatment plan, Charles hesitated: he was afraid of not being able to function, of losing control of himself and seeing his personality change. He had read on the Internet that it's not good to take drugs and that he can manage his pain himself. The team took the time to explain to him the rationale for the therapy plan; Charles then agreed to give it a try and decide on the suitability of a drug based on its results, in terms of both pain relief and general well-being.

this means that for pain management to be fully effective it must involve not just specialized health care professionals, but also patients themselves; they must play a major role in managing all pain-related symptoms, whether they are physical, emotional or cognitive. In a way, pain can be compared to a fingerprint: it's completely different from one person to the next, and each kind of pain has its own characteristics, depending on the type of damage causing it, its context, the socio-cultural baggage and psychological characteristics of the sufferer, and individual differences in metabolism and response to medication. As a result, we can't expect to overcome a challenge like chronic pain while remaining uninvolved in the suggested treatment plan. Instead, people in pain must get involved and explore complementary therapeutic approaches that might help them toward a better quality of life.

If you are someone who has to cope daily with chronic pain, the simple fact that you are reading this book shows you want to play a more active role in improving your situation. If this is so, then we believe the book has an encouraging message for you, for it is possible to better control pain and to adapt to it. While chronic pain cannot usually be cured, you can nonetheless learn to manage it and reduce its negative impact on your life by adopting a proactive multidisciplinary approach drawing on the combined knowledge of experts on pain — health care professionals, but also yourself! No specialist knows more about pain than a person who has to live with it daily.

In Summary

- Pain treatment follows a multidisciplinary assessment.

- Certain beliefs — the fear of losing control, no longer recognizing ourselves, or becoming dependent — can limit the scope of a proposed medical treatment plan. This must be discussed to ensure the best possible pain management.

- Medication, when taken as prescribed and in a responsible way, is an essential therapeutic option to consider.

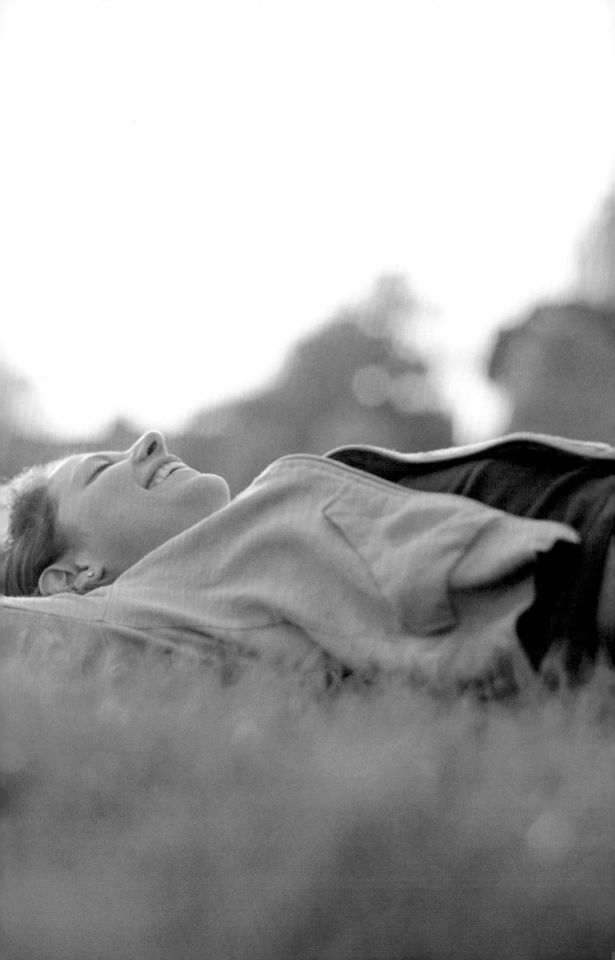

CHAPTER 6

Pain Self-Management

Experience is not what happens to man;
it is what a man does with what happens to him.

— ALDOUS HUXLEY

The whirlwind of physical and emotional hardships experienced by patients dealing with chronic pain is an unsettling experience, with many negative repercussions for psychological well-being. In the short term, these repercussions are understandable; no one can meekly accept having to cope with declining physical abilities, seeing various aspects of their social and professional life fall apart, or being forced to mourn the demise of some long-planned projects. The fear, anger and sadness felt in the face of these situations are normal — we might even say essential — emotions that must be expressed freely if the sufferer is to absorb the shock. In the longer term, however, these emotional upsets can become a trap that closes on people, imprisoning them in a vicious circle where pain darkens every aspect of their lives and leads to a significant deterioration in personality and quality of life.

One of the main challenges in treating chronic pain, therefore, is to limit these unhelpful thoughts and emotions to the shortest time period possible, so as to help people turn the page on this dark episode. At that point, it's essential to begin the recovery process, during which sufferers will acquire the necessary skills to better manage pain on a daily basis.

PERSONAL RESOURCES

The emotional response to events like mourning, job loss, illness, or unhappy love affairs can plunge people into a state where the extent of the suffering caused by these difficulties totally disrupts their lives, making them feel they have "hit bottom." The intensity and duration of these periods of distress can vary considerably depending on the individual and the nature of the challenges that must be dealt with, but in every case these periods of great vulnerability are a critical stage, a turning point in the recovery process. To regain a satisfactory quality of life, patients have to draw on personal resources to get out of this impasse, for if it lasts too long it will have serious consequences, such as depression and suicidal thoughts.

For people coping with chronic pain, returning to a normal life must involve relieving pain and eliminating its grip on all day-to-day activities. However, as we have said throughout this book, this kind of relief doesn't come from relying exclusively on painkilling medications or other medical interventions; medicine, essential though it is, has its limitations and usually can't control the pain sensation all on its own. Chronic pain relief requires holistic management targeting all of the physical, emotional, cognitive, and behavioural factors at play. In other words, to overcome the challenge of chronic pain,

The Psychological Goals of Therapy

- Improve the quality of life of the chronic pain sufferer.

- Diminish the suffering associated with depression, anxiety, and anger.

- Help sufferers sleep better and develop healthier lifestyle habits, like a balanced diet and regular physical exercise.

we have to call on our personal resources, thoughts, and emotions and learn to channel them so that they can help us cope with our pain.

The first reaction of many people to this psychological approach is disbelief: "I really do have back pain; it's not in my head; why should I work on myself?" While pain is certainly not a mental construct, psychological self-work can considerably improve

THE CURVE OF EMOTIONS AND CHRONIC PAIN

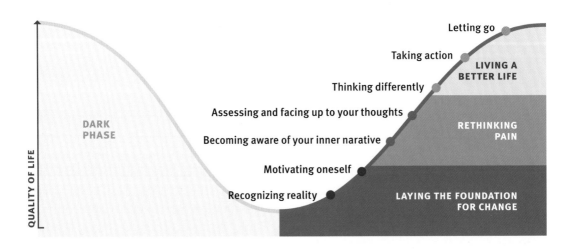

FIGURE 37

Adapted from Couture, 2010

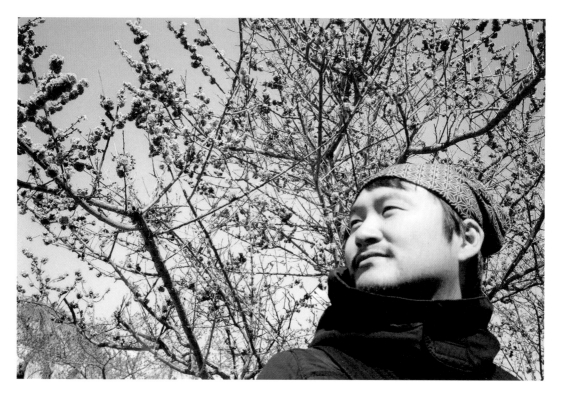

people's quality of life by reducing the intensity with which they perceive the pain and promoting a feeling of control over their pain and their lives.

This psychological approach must not be seen as a substitute for a medical approach, but rather as a complement to it. The objective of the psychological treatments discussed in this chapter is first to lessen the disruption caused by the pain so that sufferers learn to adapt to it gradually and eventually lower its perceived intensity. They are then able to regain control of their lives.

The magnitude of the challenge posed by chronic pain often means that people can't seem to identify the concrete actions they have to take to improve their situation. This hesitation is completely normal; there's no universal "recipe" for getting used to pain and each of us has to come to

terms with a unique situation as best we can. However, since adapting to all kinds of chronic pain first requires a change in thinking, a psychological approach is essential if the recovery process is to begin. This recovery process can be roughly divided into three main stages: laying the foundations for change, rethinking pain, and living a better life (Figure 37).

LAYING THE FOUNDATIONS FOR CHANGE

Laying a solid foundation for this recovery process is important. Two perspectives are especially important for getting off to a good start on the road back to a more normal life.

First of all, we must recognize the reality and acknowledge that we have chronic pain. Adapting to a situation necessarily

STAGES OF CHANGE

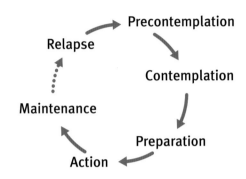

Stage of change	Meaning	Questions to ask yourself in proceeding from one stage to the next
1. Precontemplation	The person doesn't express any intention of changing and, when the subject is raised, doesn't recognize any need to change and refutes any argument in favour of change.	**Raising doubts** What are the risks or problems I might have if I don't increase my physical activity level? What are the risks for my pain and myself of not being very active?
2. Contemplation	The person indicates a desire to change to improve his or her situation. e.g.: "I could try to walk more often."	**Tipping the scale toward change** What would walking more do for me? In what way would walking be a good activity for me?
3. Preparation	The person makes a spoken commitment to make a change soon. e.g.: "I'm going to start walking twice a week, starting next week."	**Establishing a detailed plan for change** When am I going to start this walking training program? What is my goal? How well do I think I can succeed?

FIGURE 38   Based on Kerns, 1997; DiClemente and Prochaska, 1982

Stage of change	Meaning	Questions to ask yourself in proceeding from one stage to the next
4. Action	The person has been changing and modifying his or her behaviours for some time. e.g.: "I have been walking twice a day for six months now ... and I like it!"	**Making sure to be active and stay active** What have I been getting out of this walking training up to now? What would it take for me to keep doing this in the future? How has my pain been since I've started walking regularly?
5. Maintenance	The changes are ongoing, maintained over time, and have become part of the person's routine.	**Taking stock of progress** What have I accomplished up to now? How proud of myself am I? To what extent is this accomplishment important to me? Do I feel any less pain? Is my body in better shape than it was? How do I feel since I've been more active?
6. Relapse	The person abandons the behavioural change that had become routine.	**Accepting that relapse is normal and part of the change process** Why have I stopped walking? Are there benefits to me in having stopped? How is my pain since I stopped? And my quality of life? Would there be benefits for me if I started walking again?

means becoming aware of reality, and then showing a desire to adapt to it as well as possible. The first step in the pain adaptation process is thus to take stock of the situation, to admit that the pain is there and that it has consequences in our lives. This realization may seem obvious to an outside observer; after all, this is the situation these people will be in from now on; they have no choice! However, people frequently refuse to accept the new reality imposed by pain, preferring to ignore the upheavals it causes by trying to convince themselves that it's all just temporary and the pain will simply disappear, like magic. It's much harder than we might think to face up to reality, to accept that nothing will ever be quite like it was before. This process of facing reality is essential, since it allows people to see the extent of the changes they will have to make in their behaviours, thinking, and emotions, if they want to succeed in regaining the best quality of life possible. But accepting doesn't mean being resigned! Instead, it means choosing to mobilize our inner resources to cope with the pain.

Secondly, we have to motivate ourselves to change. Motivation plays a major role in adapting to pain, because no self-work can be started without a sincere desire to change. And changing is hard. Many people are deeply rooted in their habits and are reluctant to change their way of life, even when it's no longer compatible with their decreased abilities. However, change doesn't necessarily mean that everything we were doing before was not appropriate; it means that if we are dealing with chronic pain that disrupts our life, can no longer take pleasure in life, or are constantly angry, it's in

our interest to change some aspects of our lifestyle to increase enjoyment or reduce anger. Changing means we have to try to understand better what's happening in our lives so we can adapt appropriately.

Motivation to change shows in our actions: If we really want to improve our situation but don't change our habits and way of thinking in the slightest, our wish will never come true. Being motivated means taking concrete action, believing that change will be beneficial and lead to a positive outcome. Even if we have trouble believing in this at first, we have to adopt an open-minded attitude, give change a chance, and pay attention to the ensuing results.

The first stage is to figure out what has to change. Some people resist change, others are quite willing to try but only under certain conditions, and still others will let nothing stand in the way of making the desired change. What differentiates these people and, more especially, what can be done to facilitate change when it's deemed necessary?

To illustrate this process, let's take the example of someone with knee pain who has stopped doing any physical activity for fear of making the pain worse. Given his attending physician's firm insistence that he get more exercise, by walking daily, for example, he's going to have to change his habits. To do this, he will have to go through six major stages (Figure 38).

The basic principle underlying this process is to determine what will make people change their habits and then adapt their behaviour to their new abilities. Beginning to change therefore means taking time to reflect on the advantages and positive impacts this will have on their life. The more personal the reasons to change — specific to the person and directly related to individual needs — the greater the likelihood that this change will occur and really have a positive impact. But we mustn't expect to see these changes happen instantaneously! People who are afraid of moving and who have been inactive for a long time will find it hard to change their physical routines from one day to the next; they will have to change their habits gradually, one step at a time, and manage to maintain these changes for a period of time before thinking about moving on to the next stage. This gradual approach will ensure that the desired changes are realistic and suitable for their situation, while at the same time promoting a sense of success and accomplishment that boosts self-confidence.

RETHINKING PAIN

The fact that people have accepted pain as an unavoidable reality in their lives and have expressed the desire to overcome this challenge doesn't mean they've already succeeded in adapting to it, however. They also have to redefine their approach to the problem by adopting a way of thinking compatible with this new perspective, one that will positively influence their emotions and behaviours.

As we saw in Chapter 4, thoughts, emotions, and behaviours constantly interact and influence each other (Figure 39). This interaction means that we can have a direct effect on the emotional impact of pain by using that most powerful of human weapons: our ability to think.

There are three stages that have to be gone through to successfully work on our thoughts: becoming aware of our self-talk; assessing and confronting our thoughts; thinking differently.

BECOMING AWARE OF OUR SELF-TALK
We spend most of our time thinking, whether consciously or not. This internal monologue is constantly playing in our head; it's the inaudible "little voice" that "talks" to us when we are thinking or when we remember a conversation with a friend; it's the one we can hear when we talk to ourselves, often to give ourselves courage to cope with a challenge ("Come on, you can do it!"). These thoughts are sometimes very down to earth, such as when we ask

A TRIAD: THOUGHTS,
EMOTIONS, BEHAVIOURS

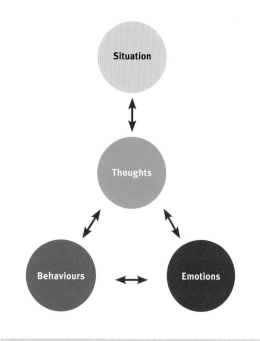

FIGURE 39

Maureen, 24

Maureen hurt her ankle badly in a work accident. Despite successful surgery and several physiotherapy treatments, she still has severe pain more than eighteen months after the accident. Maureen didn't know what to do while waiting for the pain to decrease so she could go back to work. After having felt depressed for several months, frustrated at seeing her life limited to attending medical appointments, Maureen understood that she was on the wrong track: she was much too young to give up her dreams and settle for just watching time go by. Her reflection on the meaning of her life and what she wanted to accomplish made her realize that waiting for a more effective drug and thinking dark thoughts about the circumstances of the accident were actually fear reactions — fear of coming to terms with a different life and making major changes she hadn't planned for. Aware of her limits, but also of her strengths, Maureen set herself some goals and went back to school. The pain is still there, but she has successfully adapted her new life to her physical condition, instead of letting pain control her life.

Nicole, 48

Nicole underwent a triple coronary bypass five years ago and occasionally still has very intense thoracic pain. Despite this pain, Nicole persisted in doing her usual activities, but she became irritable and depressed. The recommendations of several specialists were unequivocal: "You are doing too much! You have to pay more attention to your physical limitations!" Nicole was insulted by this: "As if my pain was in my head! What good will it do for me to change my way of thinking?" In the end she realized the comments were right: no one was telling her that her pain was imaginary, but that she had to learn to adapt to it. Once Nicole began to really listen to these comments, she agreed to modify her habits and began to feel better.

ourselves what we're going to have for dinner, and sometimes much more profound — when we feel uneasy in a particular situation, for example. Self-talk, however, is always the tangible expression of our thinking, the reflection of the brain's assessment of our current situation.

Since it's not pain per se that causes emotions, but actually thoughts — what we say to ourselves when we think about

the pain — we must become aware of this self-talk and decide whether it's compatible with improving our situation. In other words, are our spontaneously occurring thoughts really helpful?

By ourselves, it's sometimes hard to recognize thoughts that arise spontaneously in certain situations and the emotions associated with them. To become aware of the main characteristics of emotion-related self-talk, you have to really want to understand it, keeping an open mind and paying special attention to thoughts that are expressed very quietly or following a particular event. When these thoughts arise, you have to pause and once more become aware of your self-talk in order to analyze it.

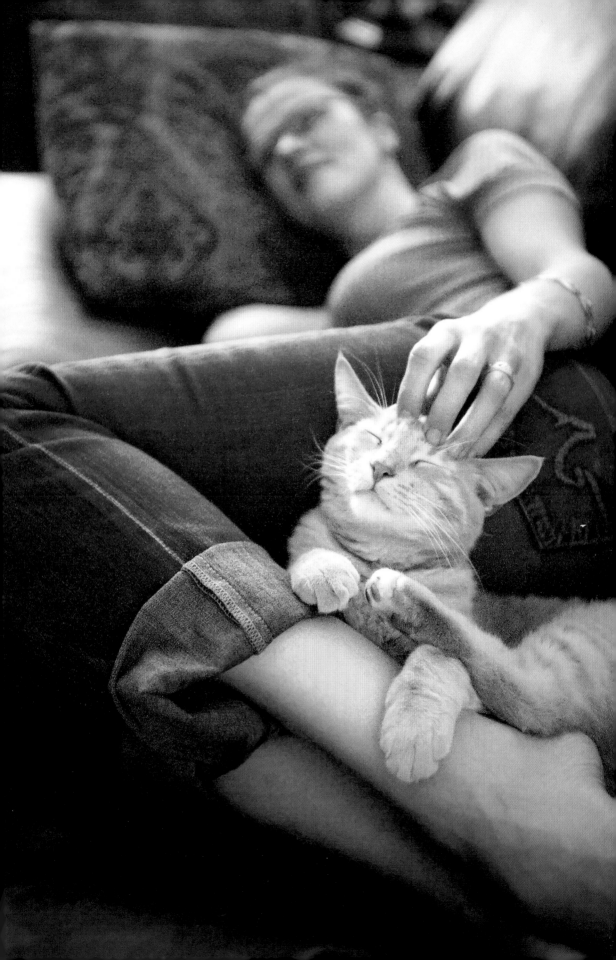

Awareness of self-talk is very important, since each of us is fully responsible for the emotions we feel in a particular situation.

ASSESSING AND CONFRONTING YOUR THOUGHTS

To ensure that your thoughts are as helpful as possible, you have to change the content of your internal monologue to make the emotions expressed more positive. This means you have to challenge your thoughts and analyze them, not to decide if they are good or bad, but rather to figure out what it is about them that's beneficial or harmful. It's not a matter of putting on rose-coloured glasses or indulging in what's known as positive or magical thinking, which often prevents us from facing up to reality by using ready-made maxims that usually don't correspond to what we are experiencing. It's useless to say that everything is fine when this is clearly not the case! Reorganizing your thoughts really means analyzing without a filter the way you approach a situation and then calling into question these ways of thinking if they negatively influence our emotions and actions. The dice are not cast at birth: fortunately, we can all change throughout our lives and adopt new behaviours by modifying our way of thinking.

Reorganizing our thoughts is crucial, because in a chronic pain context thoughts are frequently associated with various fears that not only lead to anxiety, but can also bring on depression.

Fear of Losing What We Have

Chronic pain is often accompanied by self-talk focused on the threat the pain represents both for life right now and for future plans. We are afraid of losing a job, being rejected by family or friends, or losing our freedom. In short, we lose hope with regard to our identity and life in general. Yet, although a decline in physical abilities can indeed effectively stop people from performing their activities like they used to, these fears give a false image of the reality they must face. Even if their physical capacities are different, people still have their faculties and can make a number of adjustments so as to remain self-sufficient, or, when this isn't possible, develop new interests to replace the activities hindered by pain and physical limitations. We can't define ourselves and our self-worth only by what we do. People in pain remain fundamentally the same; their personalities remain unchanged and their friends and family will still enjoy being with them. For example, there would be no reason for a woman who can no longer go fishing with her son to think of herself as a bad mother; the parameters of her interaction with the child are perhaps changed by pain, but the love she feels and gives her son remains intact and indispensable to their mutual self-fulfilment. This mother has to adapt to her current abilities to ensure she will always be able to give him this love, and in the future she will be able to count on the child's support, as the child will adapt without difficulty to the new parameters.

Fear of the Future

Uncertainty about future events is part of life. In fact, even though we really enjoy planning for the future and imagining what's going to happen (our obsession with weather forecasts is a good example), we know that there is no way to know what will happen in five minutes or five days, let alone five months. This uncertainty can become hard to live with, especially when our body is in pain and losing its abilities and we feel discouraged. People living through this therefore come to fear the future and have trouble accepting the fact that they don't know what will happen to them later on.

It's impossible to predict how our pain will evolve and it's completely understandable that we should be worried: pain can go away by itself a few months or years after its onset, remain constant, or get worse with time. What is certain, however, is that it's here *now* and is a concrete problem that must be managed. Fear of the future consequences of pain is usually just a reflection of the difficulty you are having in adapting to the present moment and finding solutions to the problems that arise in your day-to-day life. One way to accept the uncertainty about what your pain will feel like down the road and take an optimistic view of the future is to focus on the present by adopting a pragmatic approach. Several tools and strategies described in the following pages will help you stay focused on the present moment and in so doing avoid the fear, anxiety, and discouragement that can arise when we let our thoughts drift toward the future.

We must, therefore, successfully modify this self-talk, which contributes nothing useful and only makes the situation worse. While it's normal to be shattered by a sudden illness, it's nonetheless possible to limit the damage by making sure our self-talk — our way of thinking — is appropriate, realistic, and beneficial. To do this, we must first put things into perspective. Many of the events that happen to us in our

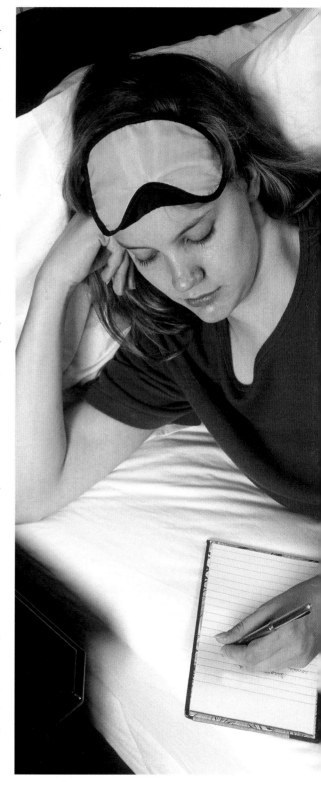

lives have little direct power over us. It's more our perception of these events and our assessment of their scope that determines their influence on us. In other words, we have the power to perceive events in a beneficial and satisfying way, or, on the contrary, in a way that is harmful, depending on the nature of our thoughts. Our assessments of tragic situations and how we react to them will determine our ability to overcome these hardships.

Coping with Situations

This power does however impose certain responsibilities. While we are in no way responsible for the cause of the events at the root of the pain, we nonetheless have the responsibility of coping with their consequences. For example, someone who has had a car accident that has left him with neuropathic pain in the legs isn't necessarily responsible for the accident, but since he's the victim, he's the only one responsible for the way he copes with the situation. Events like this truly are tragedies and extremely hard to accept, and it's normal to feel rebellious and to have strong feelings of injustice. Nonetheless, we have to find a way to get over our rebellion if we hope to regain a better quality of life. Life is full of events we have to live with, and it's our responsibility to learn to manage them as best we can or, when necessary, by seeking outside help. In the face of a life-changing situation we did not choose, the first question we have to ask ourselves, therefore, is not why pain is going to be part of our life from now on, but rather what the solutions to this problem are. Asking the following questions can help us face up to these thoughts and find an alternative way of thinking.

- What are the advantages and disadvantages of thinking this way?
- What does this thinking do for me?
- Am I happy with how I feel?

THE PYRAMID OF VALUES

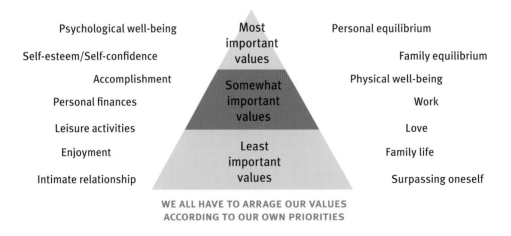

WE ALL HAVE TO ARRAGE OUR VALUES
ACCORDING TO OUR OWN PRIORITIES

FIGURE 40

142

- Why do I have these thoughts?
- What's happening to me?
- Do I recognize myself? Does this way of thinking feel like me?

It's equally important to ask ourselves questions about the relevance and realism of our various fears, given the changes caused by pain.

- What am I afraid of?
- If what I fear happened, how would it bother me?
- What's the worst that could happen to me?

By finding responses to these questions, we can make genuine contact with the self-talk we don't normally tend to examine, analyze and confront.

THINKING DIFFERENTLY

Once we've completed the stage of identifying our thoughts and asked ourselves whether or not they need to be modified, we have to find alternative thoughts that, while still realistic, will enable us to solve the problems facing us and help us regain a better quality of life. A number of important elements must be considered: fundamental values, life goals, a balanced life, the sense of self-efficacy.

Fundamental Values

Our personal values are the moral principles we live by; they influence most of our actions and choices. To restructure our thinking in a useful way, we have to take the time to revisit these values and make sure they are still in line with the changes in our lifestyle imposed by chronic pain (Figure 40). People who have spent the

Natalie, 40

Natalie suffers from knee pain after having fallen off a bicycle six years ago. Feeling depressed, she went to see a psychologist. She told him she was waiting for a meeting with the surgeon to assess the need for another operation. Natalie has already had two operations that have given her back her mobility, but without relieving her pain. The wait, which seems interminable but on which she's pinning all her hopes for relief, means that she has given up many activities: she no longer works, nor plays any sports. She was asked questions that uncovered thoughts she was not aware of: What if the surgeon told her she couldn't be operated on again? And what if she had to learn to live with her situation? She had neither thought about nor wanted to think about this possibility. She had been counting entirely on the operation. She couldn't imagine working and she believed she was the victim of an injustice since she shouldn't have to be in such pain. These thoughts had a major impact on her morale, making her discouraged and anxious. This first stage of identifying self-talk has been very revealing for her. By becoming aware of it, she has understood that she needs to examine her thinking to make sure it's realistic and, even more importantly, helpful.

CONFRONTING AND RESTRUCURING YOUR THOUGHTS

THOUGHTS	EMOTIONS	CHALLENGING YOUR THOUGHTS	NEW THOUGHTS
This can't have happened to me. / I should have been more careful. / Why is this happening to me?	Anger	Should I have been more careful? / Does getting angry make my pain worse?	I can't change anything about what happened, but what can I learn from it?
I'd rather live with another disease than this one. / I want so much to be like everybody else, without pain!	Longing	Is it possible and realistic to exchange pain for another illness? Do I usually tend to be jealous of other people?	I have to learn to live with this illness and not a different one. / How can I adapt to it as well as possible?
I can no longer help around the house like I want to; my spouse has to work twice as hard. / I can't play football with my children anymore; I'm no longer a good father.	Guilt	Is it true that I can no longer help in any way? How are these thoughts helpful? / Is it true I'm no longer a good father — in any way at all?	What can I do that's within my abilities and is helpful? / What other activity can I do with my children?
At family gatherings, I don't have anything to talk about anymore, since I don't do anything worthwhile. / Look at me, I can't walk normally anymore and I'd rather not leave the house.	Shame	Can I still offer my opinion in a conversation? Can I still listen to other people? / I don't walk the way I used to, that's true: but can I get used to it? Can I find solutions to help me?	I'm going to stay as up to date as possible on current events. I'm going to have interests and develop passions so I can talk about them.
If I'm having trouble walking at 42, what will it be like when I'm 60? / If I can't go back to work, we'll have to sell the house, because we won't be able to manage financially.	Fear of the future	Can I plan ahead for various scenarios right now, in case at 60 I can't walk anymore? / Can I examine my financial situation realistically and come up with possible solutions if, indeed, my income goes down?	Every problem has a solution! I can have confidence in my resources to manage situations as they occur. For now, I'll focus on the present moment.
As soon as I turn my head, I feel a sharp pain, so it's better not to move too much. / I've done what you told me to do, but I can't be any more active, it hurts too much.	Fear of moving	What are the advantages of not moving anymore? Is the pain less acute? / What are the disadvantages of not moving? I'll get stiffer, I'll go on being afraid, I'll be less and less active and I might get depressed.	I'm going to become more active, because I know my body has to move. I'm going to respect my limits. I'm going to challenge my fear by moving around. This is the best way to get going.

FIGURE 41

THOUGHTS	EMOTIONS	CHALLENGING YOUR THOUGHTS	NEW THOUGHTS
I prefer not to talk about my accident, not even to think about it, it's too upsetting.	Fear (PTSD)	Is it possible that not talking about it might actually increase my anxiety? Could I talk about it with a professional?	I've lived through a traumatizing experience and I need professional help; there are specialists who will be able to help me and I'm going to go out and get this help.
I'm suffocating in my house. It's as if everyone was looking at me and wondering if I'm really in pain or if I'm imagining it.	Panic	Is it normal to feel like I'm suffocating in my own house? Is there anything I could change there? Why is what others might be thinking more important than my own experience?	It's high time I learned to distance myself a little more from what others might think of me. What do I think about me? Am I imagining my pain? I'm going to try to find peace of mind with regard to other people's comments.
I cry a lot. I can't help it	Sadness	It's true, the situation is sad and I have the right to cry. Am I crying too often? Is this normal behaviour for me? Is crying in any way constructive for me?	I'm giving myself time to cry and then I'm moving on to other things. I'm keeping busy, I'm enjoying myself, and I'm finding a meaning in my life.
This is the fifth drug I've tried. There's nothing I can do, I'm still in pain.	Disappointment	It is indeed disappointing, but do I want to stop trying medications or continue as long as possible? What might I gain if I keep trying?	I can give myself the opportunity to try still other drugs, maybe one of them will help me a little. I'm going to try other strategies to manage my pain and not put all my eggs in one basket.
Even though I've tried everything, I'm still in pain. I don't know what to do.	Discouragement	Have I really tried everything? What could I do to help myself and improve my quality of life? Can I ask for help?	I think it's time I really learned to live with my pain. If 20 percent of the population lives with chronic pain, there must be someone who can give me some tips.
I've had it. I want this pain to end, even though I still love being alive.	Despair	Is there even a glimmer of hope left? What can I do to find a glimmer of hope?	I can't remain in despair. I'm going to find something to hang onto, because I want to keep on living.
I don't know what to do to help myself.	Powerlessness	Does it help me to think like this? What are the advantages and disadvantages?	I think I've tried everything by myself; now I'm going to consult a professional who will know how to help me.

greater part of their time working and are obliged to put a halt to their professional activities because of pain must by necessity review the importance they placed on work, to avoid sinking into a deep depression. Too many people base their self-esteem on what they do and not on who they are. This reflects our society's strong emphasis on performance and the

Advice to Help Set Goals

Here are a few tips to help set realistic daily or general goals.

Make sure the chosen goal is realistic.
- Can this goal be achieved in spite of pain?
- Is it beyond the person's physical capacities?
- Is it adapted to the person's physical, medical, and psychological condition?

The goal must be concrete.
- Is the purpose clear and specific?
- What are the required stages to reach this goal?
- Will it be possible to determine if it has been reached or not?

The goal must be personal.
- People have to choose their own goals, ones that are meaningful to them. They are the main players, the ones who get involved in the activity. For example, the spouses of people who set goals for themselves can't be held responsible for achieving this goal.

admiration we have for people who stop at nothing, always seeking a new challenge to overcome. These people are certainly outstanding, but so are many people who may do somewhat less.

For example, people in pain who nonetheless manage to do something at the limit of their abilities accomplish something praiseworthy and worthwhile. We thus have to take a new look at how we do things — not consider activities only from the perspective of the final result, but also take into account how the result was achieved. It's possible to paint a picture that will remain anonymous, but be very proud of it nonetheless, because it represents the accomplishment of a difficult goal that only happened because of determination to overcome limits imposed by pain.

Life Goals
Redefining a person's fundamental values is usually accompanied by changes in life goals, both short-term and longer-term. Setting goals is very important, because it keeps people from adopting a passive attitude to events and remaining petrified by the idea of having to tolerate pain over a long period of time. Keeping a very full calendar, with at least one clear goal every day — household tasks, reading, exercise, other hobbies — is a good way to do this. All activities should be listed; this will show that one's days are fully occupied and that planned activities are actually taking place. When daily routine is disrupted by pain, it becomes even more important to plan at least one enjoyable activity each day; if there are no activities planned, it's very likely that people will get to the end of the day without having

done anything. These goals must of course be based on their physical abilities. For example, being able to walk for thirty consecutive minutes can be a considerable challenge for some people. But they might manage it by establishing intermediate steps to allow them to gradually increase their mobility, and in the end reach the goal. Whatever a patient's condition, it's essential to set goals. Patients can then structure their day and get organized in a way that encourages them to accomplish activities within their limitations.

A Balanced Life

Over time, people in pain can come to feel that pain and the physical disabilities it entails have become the centre of their lives; the result can be serious psychological imbalance. They must be shown that pain is not all-important; it's just one aspect of life, among many others (Figure 42).

A Sense of Self-Efficacy

Self-efficacy encompasses all the beliefs people have about their ability to accomplish tasks or carry out activities. There are several kinds of belief: how we manage a fortunate or unfortunate event; our ability to control pain and the emotional reactions it evokes in various situations; our success in continuing to carry out daily activities (continuing to work, participating in leisure activities, communicating our needs, and asking for help when necessary). The greater the sense of self-efficacy, the better the prognosis for good pain management.

This is beyond a doubt one of the most important parameters in adapting to pain, for if people don't believe they have the necessary resources to overcome a difficulty, they have very few reasons to act or persevere when faced with hardship. A sense of self-efficacy gives them confidence in their ability to withstand pain while accomplishing a task or in a specific situation, without necessarily knowing

A BALANCED LIFE

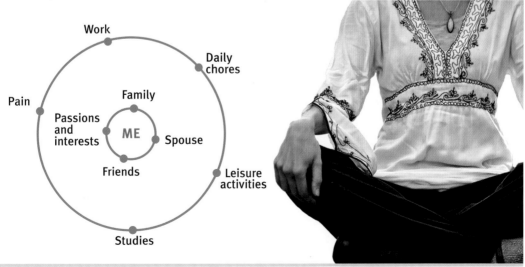

FIGURE 42

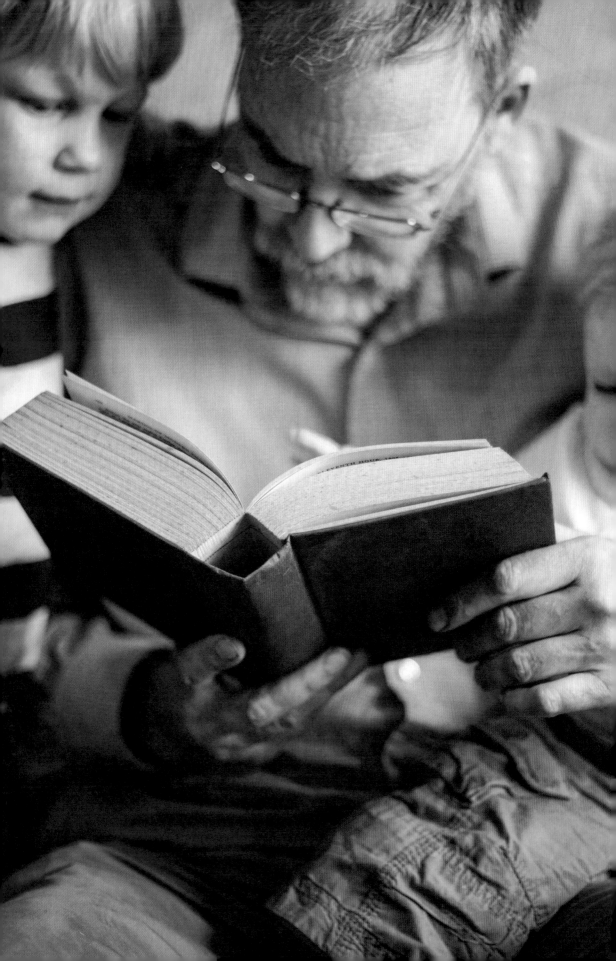

what the result of the activity will be. As set out by Albert Bandura, this concept suggests that expectations of efficacy determine how much effort people will put into overcoming an obstacle or a difficult situation.

A sense of self-efficacy can develop over time, even in people who have very little confidence in their personal resources. When people are motivated by the idea of improving their condition and begin to modify their thoughts and behaviours, their physical and psychological progress has a number of positive effects on their quality of life, which, in turn, can only enhance their confidence in their abilities. We must not, therefore, get discouraged. Even when we feel helpless to cope with chronic pain, we have to remember that everyone has inner resources that can be mobilized to deal with this challenge. If we don't already have these resources, it's perfectly possible to acquire them on our own or to get the necessary psychological help. Self-confidence is acquired and maintained by what we do. We have to nurture it by taking action.

Restructuring thoughts and behaviours can have a direct impact on emotions and thus on a person's well-being. This shows how beneficial self-work can be.

Figure 41 contains examples of the process of turning unrealistic or unhelpful thoughts into realistic, helpful, and pleasant ones. By undertaking these changes, we can have a direct influence on emotions and moderate them. For example, this work can make anger less intense and help it pass more quickly, or alleviate a fear of movement by making people more confident and more active in their daily lives, without necessarily increasing their pain.

Figure 43 summarizes a few of the strategies available to decrease the intensity of the distress associated with various psychological disorders.

LIVING A BETTER LIFE

Once you've begun to work on your thinking, it's important to take action and put yourself in situations where you can experience and apply everything you've "re-thought." You can reflect constantly, discuss and exchange ideas at length, but without actual concrete actions, nothing will happen. To feel better, achieve your goals and overcome your limitations, you have to take action.

TAKING ACTION AND FINDING A NEW DAILY ROUTINE

There's no denying that chronic pain decreases abilities and limits activities, but this doesn't mean you have to be completely passive where day-to-day tasks are concerned. It's definitely possible to get a lot done by keeping an open mind about changes that will enable you to do things differently. For example, it may no longer be possible to vacuum every room in the house one after another, but you could do one room a day. The same is true for laundry, grocery shopping, errands, and other household chores. If you can no longer do them the way you used to, you have to find a new way to get them done. It's a matter of adapting your daily routine to your abilities instead of your pain, of not thinking in terms of what you can't do and your limitations, and focusing instead on what you can do. Just because you can no longer manage to complete a task in the same way or in the

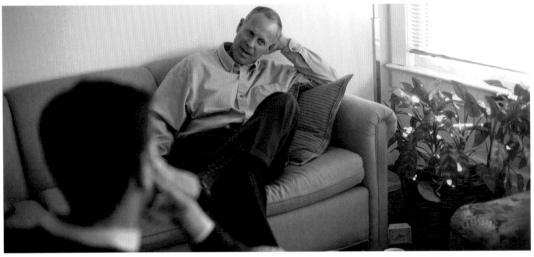

STRATEGIES FOR DEALING WITH VARIOUS PSYCHOLOGICAL PROBLEMS

Psychological disorder	Examples of strategies
Excessive anxiety	• Challenge your fears and worries. • Establish concrete and realistic steps to adopt to keep the anxiety at a manageable level. • Consult a psychologist to learn about recognized and effective treatment protocols. • Assess the option of taking medication.
Panic	• Stay calm and wait for the symptoms to decrease and then stop, as panic is not dangerous. • Stay where you are and don't run away from where you are. • Face the panic: the less you fear it, the less intense it will be and the faster your symptoms will fade. • Identify the factors that trigger it or sustain it so you can prevent it.
Agoraphobia	• Become aware of panic management strategies to increase your self-confidence. • Work on developing the necessary confidence no matter where you are or what situation you find yourself in, whether you are alone or not.

FIGURE 43

Post-traumatic stress	• See a psychologist or psychiatrist who specializes in treating this disorder.
Catastrophic thinking	• Work on modifying thoughts focusing on rumination, helplessness, or imagining the worst, and replace them with other thoughts focused on finding solutions.
	• Challenge the idea that pain is responsible for everything by performing a variety of activities and getting physically active.
	• Follow a gradual and progressive program to return to physical activity (work, physical exercises, household chores, etc.) so as to remain as active as you can.
Depression	• Ask yourself why you feel the way you do (discouraged, sad, helpless).
	• Ask yourself what you have to do or modify (small changes and big ones) to change things.
	• Remember that depression is the result of our evaluation of our pain and not the pain itself.
	• Get active so as to stimulate interest and motivation.
	• If the depression is severe and self-work is difficult, think about psychotherapy and (or) taking appropriate medication.
Suicidal thoughts	• Talk about your suicidal thoughts.
	• Share your feelings with those around you whom you trust.
	• Don't shut yourself away from people or be afraid of talking about it.
	• Immediately consult a doctor or a psychologist if suicidal thoughts persist or become hard to control.
	• When the situation becomes critical and you think you are going take concrete action, dial 911 or go to emergency at a hospital. Health professionals will help you.

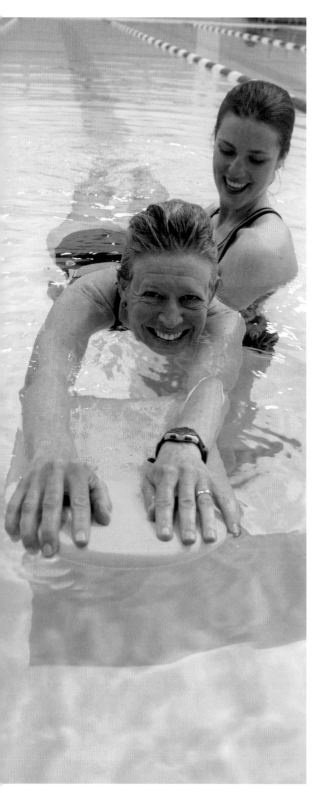

same period of time as before doesn't mean you can't derive great satisfaction from it — quite the opposite.

However, you have to learn to manage your energy and make sure the efforts you make are adapted to your physical situation, to avoid exceeding your abilities and paying the price later on. Keeping a record of the intensity of the pain at different times of day is a good way to do this: Is the pain more intense in the morning, evening, after vigorous activity? This kind of record lets you draw up a basic plan for scheduling activities. For each activity to be done, you must assess the energy required and make sure you have time to replenish your energy.

Work and Self-Fulfilment

Being active is important — through action we can find self-fulfilment. But you have to decide which kinds of activities are best suited to your current physical abilities, all the while keeping the brain and body alert. Lack of success is not a failure; it's completely normal to have to make several attempts to find your new comfort zone. For people who are able to do so, it's important to keep working as long as possible, as a professional occupation makes us feel useful and means we are contributing to the life of the community, both values that remain essential for most people. When the work environment no longer allows people in pain to function normally, it may be possible to redirect their careers toward work that corresponds to their current abilities, or perhaps to take training that will lead to an appropriate job. Volunteer work may be an attractive solution when salaried work is really no longer possible, as the satisfaction of helping someone else can be very gratifying and often helps put our own problems into perspective. It's important to focus on your current abilities and make the most of them.

Physical Exercise

The human body is meant to be active and loses its abilities during prolonged inactivity. In times past, the "good" advice given to everybody dealing with pain, like intense back pain, was to stay in bed and rest while waiting for the pain to decrease. Several studies and clinical observations done in recent years indicate, however, that this was likely the worst advice that could be given to these people! A body that moves less stiffens up, becomes less able to perform movements and, as we have seen, this loss of conditioning drags you into a downward spiral that can lead to depression or trigger catastrophic thinking. All parts of the body need to move, the painful areas just like the healthy ones. It's therefore essential to develop, together with a movement therapist, an action plan that will allow you to exercise the painful area in different ways without making the injury worse. Feeling a slight degree of pain after physical effort or exercise is normal. If this pain becomes very intense and makes you unable to function, this doesn't mean that you're unable to move, but simply that the physical exercise was not appropriate for your body in its current condition. The important thing is not to get discouraged and to continue to be active, as the right kind of activity at the right level of intensity for a particular painful condition can always be found.

Mary, 54

Mary had to stop working because of intense neuropathic pain following a mastectomy. Nonetheless, she began to do volunteer work with seniors who were losing their independence by helping two people who couldn't feed themselves two days a week and keeping them company. At first, Mary didn't think she'd be able to commit herself because her pain was sometimes unpredictable. But she gave it a try, and in three years she has seldom missed a day. Something to be proud of!

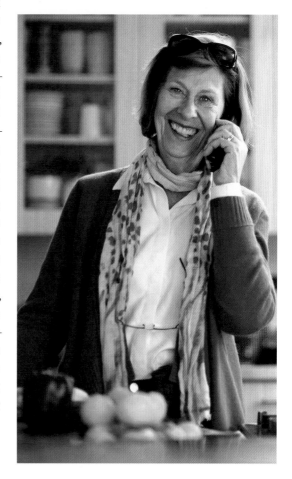

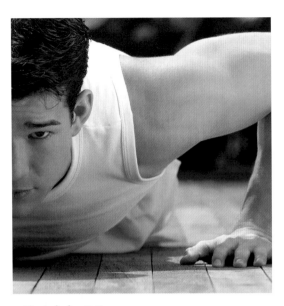

Patrick, 26

Patrick had a motorbike accident resulting in multiple fractures that have impaired his physical abilities and triggered persistent pain. Patrick realized during his stay in a rehabilitation centre that the difference between those who "make it" and those who don't lies in determination and perseverance. He had been given a medical recommendation to exercise to maintain his abilities. Since he got out, Patrick has been going to the gym four times a week, a prescription he gave himself. He isn't training to be the strongest man or to run marathons, but rather to stay in shape and keep his spirits up, and especially to limit the effect of his pain, which otherwise would be more intense and keep him from doing what he wants. He has also noticed that when he cuts back on his training sessions, his body feels it, the pain is stronger, and he has less energy and feels more tired.

Eating Well

A healthy diet is absolutely necessary; in addition to supplying the energy needed for the body to function properly, what we eat directly influences the smooth functioning of all our cells. Here are a few pieces of advice on eating better:

Fill up on plants. All plant foods, whether fruits, vegetables, whole grains, spices, or certain drinks like tea, contain significant quantities of antioxidant and anti-inflammatory molecules that have a positive influence on how the body functions. In terms of chronic pain, this anti-inflammatory action is especially interesting, for several kinds of pain are caused at least in part by prolonged inflammation. Eating more plant foods is thus a useful way to prevent excessive inflammation that could make the pain worse. These foods are still all too often ignored, but they are indispensable in maintaining good health and should have pride of place in everyone's diet, especially those who have to deal with chronic pain.

Omega-3, the king of fats. Omega-3 fatty acids are polyunsaturated fats that play a role in many cellular functions, notably the inflammatory and immune response. Fatty fish (salmon, sardines, mackerel), as well as certain plants and flax seed in particular, are major sources of omega-3, and eating them regularly (once or twice a week) is a simple and effective way to increase the benefits of these fats in our diets.

Down with bad food! Some overly-processed manufactured foods contain extraordinary quantities of sugar, fat, refined flours, and salt. This junk food is very bad for our health, as its ingredients keep our cells from functioning properly. For example, too much sugar and refined flour cause significant fluctuations in blood glucose. Over time this can create a systemic inflammatory environment that can only harm a pain sufferer. The high sugar and fat content of these foods also causes us to consume too many calories, increasing the risk of becoming overweight and obese; in turn, this excess weight makes the impact of various kinds of chronic pain worse (osteoarthritis, arthritis, carpal tunnel).

Pay attention. Paying attention to the effects of foods on the body is important, even in the case of foods deemed good for health. For example, medications can have a negative impact on bowel habits and cause unpleasant side effects during the digestion of certain classes of foods.

Simplify your life. The physical restrictions pain imposes are the main obstacle to a good diet, but a number of strategies can be put into practice to get around these limitations: prepare healthy snacks ahead of time for when you feel really hungry, prepare meals in larger quantities and freeze them so you can use them when the pain is too intense and keeps you from cooking. It really is worthwhile to use your imagination, for of all the things we do, eating well is one of the most likely to have a positive influence on the quality of life of people with chronic pain.

Sleeping Well

Sleep plays a key role in pain perception, from both a physical and psychological point of view. Be sure you have good sleeping habits.

Social Relationships

People in pain need healthy communication with friends and family and those around them to combat isolation and develop the harmonious social relationships their well-being requires. We are first and foremost social animals, and the simple fact of meeting people, talking to them and listening to them provides enjoyment and gives us something other than pain to think about.

Successfully maintaining this social network requires the mutual participation of patients and those close to them. Some patients find it extremely difficult to ask

Advice on Sleeping Well

- Set aside at least an hour to relax before bedtime.

- Only go to bed when you feel sleepy: try not to spend a lot of time in bed during the day.

- If you can't sleep, get up and leave the bedroom.

- Limit the length of daytime naps to twenty to thirty minutes.

- Sleeping on a good mattress, in a horizontal position, is still the best way to get a good night's rest. Avoid sleeping on the sofa or in a chair for long periods as this will have an impact on your sleep.

- Sleep at night and live during the day! Make sure your sleep isn't displaced into the daytime. If this is the case, look at the reasons why and try to find a solution.

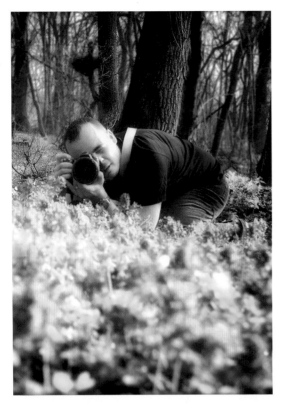

Mark, 36

Mark has had to reorganize his daily routine, since multiple sclerosis keeps him from being as active as before, as well as causing periods of pain and sometimes very intense muscular weakness. Mark was a high-performance cyclist and most of his leisure activities were centred around cycling, an activity he hasn't been able to do for several years now. However, although he thought it would be impossible, he has discovered another passion: photography. Once someone with no interest in anything but cycling, Mark has become open to other possibilities and has accepted that the choice of finding a new passion is his to make. He chose to change and now he's hooked!

for help and this reluctance often makes developing relationships of trust difficult. It's important to learn to ask and to receive, as long as you maintain a balance between what you receive and what you give to others. Giving can mean very different things for different people: even if pain has diminished our abilities, we can still make the most of our strengths or our knowledge, give love, time, listen and help. It's important for friends and family to avoid over-protecting people in pain as much as possible and not to channel the helplessness we feel when loved ones are suffering into constantly trying to do everything for them. This kind of environment prevents people in pain from taking the physical and psychological steps essential to their progress toward a better quality of life.

Leisure Activities

If you can no longer enjoy the leisure activities you used to do, you have to find new ones! Having fun is absolutely key to a balanced life. Pleasure can be found in little everyday things: reading a book on a subject you are passionate about, tasting food you like, watching a TV program, talking with or meeting someone. Above all, pleasure can (and must) be connected to the present moment.

LETTING GO

Living with chronic pain is a stressful ordeal, both physiologically and psychologically. The close relationship between body and mind has the effect of upsetting people's emotional and cognitive balance. We often notice that the body seems to exist in a state of hypervigilance, constantly on the lookout for the least sign of different or more intense pain, and fearing any situation that could make the pain worse. In short, the whole person marches to the beat of the pain, without pausing, unable to "stand easy" and let go of the stress.

Abdominal breathing, various relaxation techniques, self-hypnosis, or hypnosis give you a feeling of control over your body, soothe emotions like anxiety or anger, and alleviate pain. Several scientific studies have shown that these self-regulation techniques, practiced for thousands of years in some cultures, allow the body to effectively release accumulated tension, relax, and regain a degree of physical equilibrium. As a result, these techniques also lead to a renewed sense of well-being and inner peace.

They are not magic, however, and you mustn't expect the pain to disappear or that this feeling of well-being will be permanent or lasting. Like all pain management strategies, relaxation must be incorporated into your routine and practiced regularly for it to be truly beneficial and shorten the periods of most intense pain. Most people who practice one or several of these techniques get significant benefits from them, even those who were somewhat skeptical at the beginning. These techniques allow you to pause deliberately, to clear your mind so you can focus on being in the present moment. They cannot in any way replace the medications or other treatments needed to manage pain well, but they can nonetheless add a complementary dimension and magnify the benefits of other therapeutic approaches. Let's take a look at abdominal breathing and hypnosis.

Abdominal Breathing

Although very simple, this is the basis of all relaxation techniques. It's the deep natural breathing that we normally do during sleep

RESPIRATION

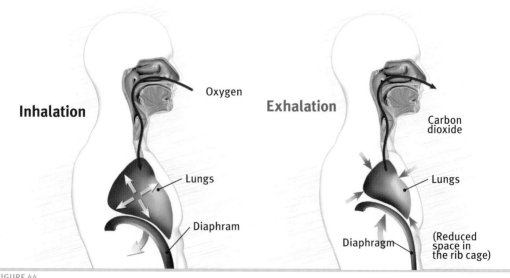

Inhalation — Oxygen — Lungs — Diaphram

Exhalation — Carbon dioxide — Lungs — Diaphragm — (Reduced space in the rib cage)

FIGURE 44

Learning to Breathe and Relax

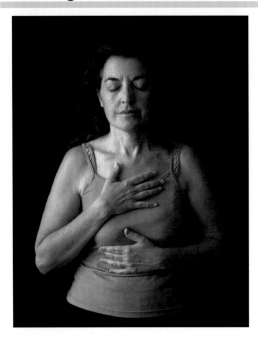

Evaluating your Breathing

Test No. 1
How many breaths do you take in sixty seconds? (A breath is one inhalation followed by an exhalation.)

Test No. 2
What part of your body moves the most when you breathe? To find out, place one hand on your chest and the other on your abdomen.

☐ Abdomen
☐ Chest

Abdominal breathing
Breathing that leads to relaxation is done with the muscles in the diaphragm, located under the rib cage. It's deep and calm, reduces the symptoms of stress and can keep them from getting worse.

Technique to try
- Place one hand on your abdomen and the other on your chest. If your chest seems to expand more than your abdomen, try blocking it by applying slight pressure.

- Inhale while counting slowly to three in your head, and then exhale slowly while repeating to yourself the word "relax" or any other word that you associate with relaxation. Inhalation and exhalation must take about six seconds. Your breathing rate should therefore be ten breaths per minute.

- Normal breathing rate should be between 10 and 14 breaths per minute (inhalation and exhalation).

- Try practicing this exercise twice a day for about ten minutes at the beginning, at times when you are calm. Later on, you'll be able to use this technique in situations you find stressful or when pain is more intense.

This technique can be practiced discreetly, quickly and wherever you like, whenever you need to regain your balance and relax.

or in moments of relaxation, and it transports oxygen throughout the body. Conversely, when we experience powerful emotions or stress, or adopt poor posture, our breathing becomes more superficial, involving only the chest and creating an imbalance between the oxygen entering the organism and the carbon dioxide given off. In the medium term, this kind of breathing can cause additional muscle tension and make us feel like we have a weight, and sometimes even pain, in the chest. Learning to breathe slowly, deeply, and regularly into the abdomen not only makes it possible to eliminate these sensations, but also to reduce anxiety and physical tension, and thus re-establish harmony in the body.

Hypnosis

The trance phenomenon has been used for many centuries. In ancient Greece, hypnosis was used to cure diseases using post-hypnotic suggestions. In the nineteenth century, surgeon James Esdaile performed several operations on patients under hypnosis. We are also familiar with

HYPNOSIS: QUESTIONS AND ANSWERS

Frequently asked questions	Answers
What can hypnosis do for me?	With hypnosis you can regain control over your life, by letting go of what is causing you problems. Letting go doesn't mean giving up, but rather directing your energy where it's needed, taking a break, and coming back to the present moment.
Can this technique really cure me?	This technique doesn't aim to cure pain, but actually to promote its relief and provide a tool for managing both physical tension and emotions.
Under hypnosis can you do things you wouldn't want to do?	In a hypnotic state, you do nothing you don't want to do.
Will the hypnotherapist take control of my brain?	The hypnotherapist in no way takes control of the hypnotized person: he or she uses techniques to suggest and guide the person toward feeling better. The person retains control at all times and decides whether or not to accept the proposed suggestion.
Who can be hypnotized?	Some people are very easy to hypnotize, others not at all. Everybody can benefit from it!
How is it different from stage hypnosis?	Stage hypnosis is used solely for amusement and very often only those easily hypnotized are chosen (when the performance isn't "fixed," of course).

FIGURE 45

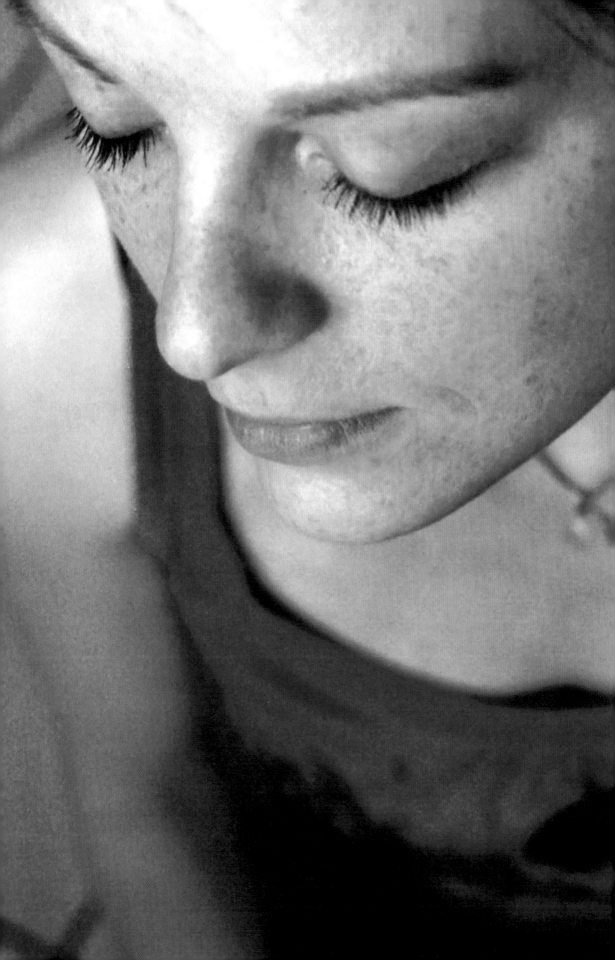

mesmerism, named after Dr. Franz-Anton Mesmer who, during hypnosis sessions with his patients, made suggestions to them while speaking to them. These techniques have remained in use, but much less since the discovery of anaesthetics. That said, in recent years hypnosis has come to be viewed as a natural process leading to an altered state of consciousness that can be highly therapeutic. Individuals have full control of what they do and are absorbed by their task while remaining oblivious to their surroundings (Figure 45).

In an altered state of consciousness, people are neither sleeping nor fully awake. They are in full control of themselves, aware of being in a kind of voluntary trance that gives them a feeling of well-being. In this state, they are more receptive to suggestions (usually spoken), are able to modify certain perceptions and memory, and can control involuntary movements. Under hypnosis, the hypnotized person remains fully in charge. In no way does anyone else (the hypnotist) take control of them. Everything done under hypnosis is done voluntarily. It's the person's ability to concentrate and imagine what is being suggested that lets them enter a hypnotic state. People under hypnosis abandon themselves to the suggestions made to them. This notion of abandonment is central, since it entails a letting go of reality, first to modify it and then to reap its benefits. For example, people who have had chronic pain for at least several months may have adopted a hypervigilant attitude and be on constant alert to avoid further injury. This puts them into a severe state of physical tension that reinforces their need to control everything outside themselves to keep from being hurt. This need for control runs counter to the idea of relaxation, rest-ing, and letting go; these people therefore have to learn to relax, minimize the importance of what's happening outside, and

Lucy, 45

Lucy has musculoskeletal back pain varying in intensity from 5 to 7 out of 10. She has good medical monitoring and takes the appropriate medications, and she gets physical exercise adapted to her capacities. However, in times of stress at work, she notes that her pain becomes more intense and harder to control. This has a negative impact on the rest of her day, causing fatigue, irritability, and discouragement. Isabelle has chosen to try a form of hypnosis, self-hypnosis, to put herself into a state where she can relax her muscles, empty her mind, and think only about the present moment. In this way, she manages to counteract the effects of stress on her body and on her pain, and gets a moment's relief while keeping her pain from getting worse. Because she practices this technique every day, Isabelle knows how to use it when the pain gets worse or during major stress. She finds this therapeutic tool effective and complementary to the other strategies she uses to manage her pain.

focus instead on what's happening inside. Hypnosis lets people pause and voluntarily and, in a healthy way, cut themselves off from their surroundings to find out what is happening inside themselves, to develop it, nurture it and explore all its possibilities in order to feel better and, in the long run, alleviate the pain. Under hypnosis, people can learn to face their pain, ask themselves why they have it, and whether they can or cannot live with it. Some people with a vivid imagination are able to visualize their pain, give it a shape or a colour, form an image of it, and then modify it as they wish. For example, a neuropathic pain experienced as a kind of burning sensation may in part be relieved by suggestions aiming to "cool down" the pain, or even by having people imagine themselves in a frigid environment on a beautiful winter's day, which would have the effect of relieving the burning sensation. Under hypnosis, you can change or modulate a sensation, perception, thought or behaviour.

Many scientific studies confirm the usefulness of hypnosis and its effectiveness in reducing chronic pain. In 1997 Pierre Rainville and his colleagues used brain imaging to show beyond a doubt that several brain structures involved in pain perception are influenced by hypnotic suggestion. Dr. Marie-Élisabeth Faymonville, who studies the phenomenon of hypnosis by means of brain imaging, uses hypnosedation in operations in Liège, Belgium. Since 1992 she has used hypnosis combined with local anaesthesia on more than six thousand patients who have undergone various major and minor operations. Dr. Faymonville maintains that this approach results in greater comfort during and after surgery, better recovery, less fatigue, and more active participation on the part of the patient. This impressive initiative attests to the effectiveness and thus the importance of hypnosis in the medical context.

When practiced regularly, these techniques for promoting rest, relaxation, self-control, and letting go can be very effective in reducing stress and tension in the body, but also in relieving pain. They complement psychological, physical, and medical treatments, and can promote a state of well-being that can sometimes be surprising. Given their effectiveness, they should be part of any treatment plan for relieving pain.

In Summary

- Psychological treatments focused on restructuring our thinking help us become aware of self-talk and its impact on emotions and show us how to modify it realistically in order to feel better.

- Changing your thinking means you can take an active part not just in your treatments, but also in your life, despite having pain.

- Practicing techniques like abdominal breathing and hypnosis can prove very effective as part of an overall treatment strategy for chronic pain.

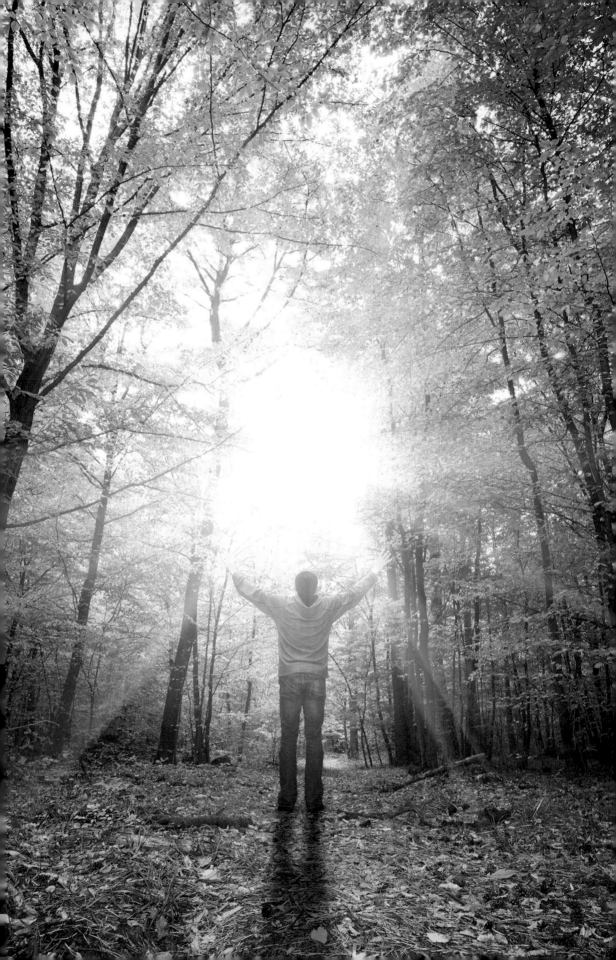

Cultivating Greater Well-Being

These are several easy-to-remember ways to keep you from becoming discouraged if your pain becomes more intense and you have to get through a difficult period.

STAY CALM

Worrying and imagining the worst will not help the situation at all. It will actually have the effect of creating physical stress that can increase pain and prevent you from thinking clearly and finding a solution.

BE AWARE OF THE TOOLS AND STRATEGIES AVAILABLE TO YOU

Even if the pain becomes very intense and some tools don't seem to work, don't get discouraged. These tools are still useful and you won't lose the ability to use them; it's just harder at the moment to use them to manage your pain. They will be effective again once the pain returns to its normal intensity. If some of these tools are usually more effective, they can be the most useful in more difficult moments.

USE RELAXATION STRATEGIES

The more you use these techniques in good times, the more useful they will be when pain strikes. Don't forget that by taking a few seconds to stop and practise abdominal breathing, you send a message to your body that you are quietly taking back control.

TALK TO YOUR FRIENDS AND FAMILY

People close to you, who live with you or regularly spend time with you, can be very helpful. You have the right to ask them for assistance to make things easier for you. These people, if they know you well, will also be able to help you find ways to better manage your pain attacks. Stay in touch with people as much for the support they can offer in bad times as in good times.

FIND ENJOYABLE THINGS TO DO

Remember that enjoyable activity is a powerful painkiller. Stay as busy as possible, while always being aware of your current abilities. Remain as active as you can, but if the pain is very intense and considerably limits your activities, choose more passive ways of having fun, like watching a movie or a TV show.

TALK TO YOUR DOCTOR ABOUT RE-EVALUATING YOUR MEDICATION

Over time, the pain may not respond as well to your medications and can become harder to manage. Your doctor can reassess the pain and decide if there are other factors (illness, stress, depression) that are having a negative impact on the effectiveness of your medication. This kind of review with your doctor can be a big help to you in laying out a new game plan.

MAKE A LIST

In your most difficult moments, it can be very hard to think and see clearly. Plan ahead! Make a list of everything that could help you at those times. For example, you could post in a strategic room in your house a list of activities to do depending on the pain's intensity, people to contact for help, or effective strategies to help you enjoy yourself.

STAY ACTIVE

Remember that it's very important, even in periods of intense pain, to remain as active as possible. Make walking a priority, even if you don't go as far or as fast as usual. Most importantly, get your body moving — don't let pain take over.

TAKE THE "PULSE" OF YOUR EMOTIONS

It's perfectly normal to be depressed, discouraged, or angry when pain becomes more intense and harder to control. But if you stay that way for more than a few hours, the situation will just get worse. If you feel you are losing control not only of your pain, but also of your emotions and state of mind, talk to a loved one or your doctor, or see a psychologist who will be able to help you regain control.

PREPARE YOURSELF PSYCHOLOGICALLY

Difficult moments will recur — it's normal. Pain can sometimes vary for reasons we know or for others we can't explain. Have confidence in yourself. Make use of all the tools you now have within your reach. Don't let pain take you by surprise. Even when you are in pain, if it gets worse, either tackle it head on or do what you have to do to fight it, control it or simply co-exist with it.

JOIN A SUPPORT GROUP

Chronic pain is a solitary ordeal and it can be very comforting to share your experiences, both positive and negative, with other people in a similar situation.

Learning to Live Differently

Our bodies are our gardens, to which our wills are gardeners.
— William Shakespeare, *Othello*

The search for happiness is a fundamental characteristic of the human soul, the driving force that enables us to overcome the many trials that confront us during our lives. While this ability to cope with adversity, to roll with the punches and make an even stronger comeback later on, exists in each of us, it's by no means automatic; being content or feeling happy are not states that can be achieved without a large investment of energy and a fervent desire to improve our condition. In the face of unfair or cruel events that occur without warning and upset our lives, we have to rally all our resources to regain control and find renewed happiness.

Being able to rally resources is especially important for people living with chronic pain. As we have seen throughout this book, living with persistent pain is a demanding ordeal, not only because of the physical limitations it imposes, but

also because it affects the entire person and profoundly disrupts every sphere of life. The challenge of chronic pain is all the greater because generally it can neither be cured nor completely alleviated. Faced with a challenge of this magnitude, sufferers must above all rely on themselves, on their ability to draw on all of their personal resources to adapt successfully to their new condition and find renewed enjoyment in life. To be confronted with chronic pain is to be confronted with oneself. It means realizing that despite the burden imposed by the pain, we remain solely responsible for our lives and well-being.

While we can't cure chronic pain, we can nonetheless "rethink" this illness and modify our way of dealing with it by developing mental and emotional skills that reduce the pain's intensity and its negative effects on daily life. This is an extremely

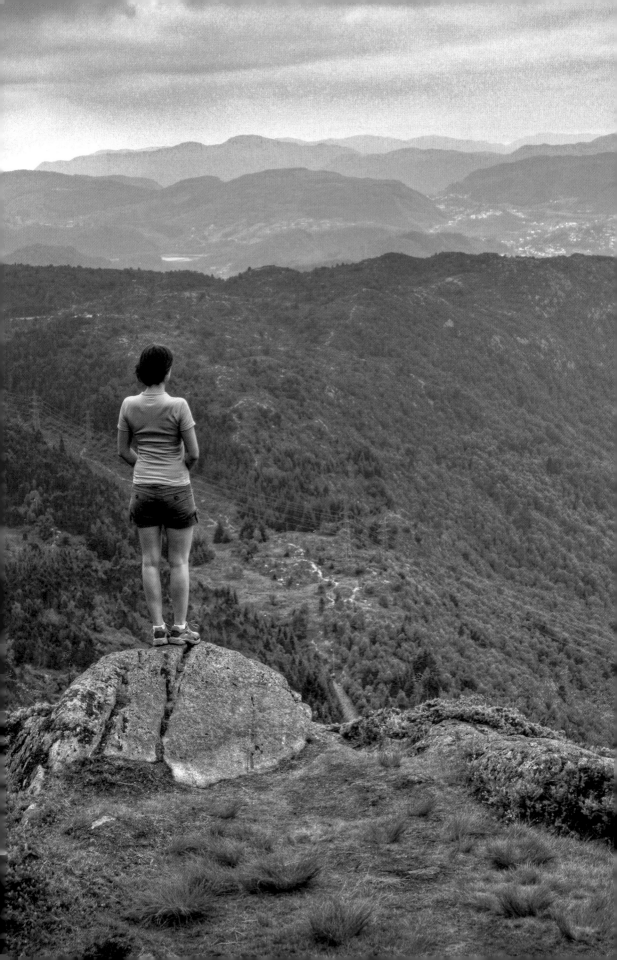

important concept: people coping with chronic pain are not as powerless as they might think, even when medical intervention doesn't provide the hoped-for results. As we have discussed in this book, there are a number of tools and strategies that can help change how we approach pain, so as to adapt to it and enhance our quality of life. These tools must not be viewed as a miracle recipe that we just have to put into practice without too much thought in order to live a better life; instead these are general principles that we can all apply to own experience, character, and the circumstances of the challenge we are dealing with. The most important thing is to be open to the problem of pain and accept that from now on it will be part of our life, but to tell ourselves that it still doesn't have to become the centre of our existence to the detriment of our well-being.

As someone with chronic pain, you must become your own pain expert, for you know better than anyone else what you feel and how effective the strategies used to fight the illness you are dealing with are. First, you have to find your own motivation, which is unique to each of us. For some, love for children and spouse will be the main motivation, while for others, it might be going back to work or changing careers to discover a new sense of accomplishment. Of course, this also requires a change in lifestyle habits, reviewing your way of thinking, and making sure you do your part "actively" to enhance your own physical and psychological well-being.

For people with chronic pain, managing to overcome this challenge is a source of great pride, both because of the improved quality of life and the discovery of a courage and resilience they did not suspect they possessed. It's not unusual for them to emerge from this fight completely transformed, with some even feeling that redefining their lives and their priorities has made them better people, more balanced, and more emotionally stable. It's therefore possible to find meaning in pain, to view this situation not only from the perspective of what has been lost, but also as a constructive challenge that lets us express the best of ourselves in an enhanced relationship with our surroundings. This kind of accomplishment is within everyone's grasp.

We are convinced that instead of having a passive attitude toward pain and waiting for an imminent medical miracle that will cure all ills, it's possible to react positively, to get the most out of medical treatments, both physical and psychological, to adopt an assertive attitude that will help us master pain and better control its impact on our daily lives as a result. As with all difficulties in life, the most formidable weapon for coping with this challenge is located within ourselves, in the amazing ability we have to adapt to the worst events and come out winners, still driven by the irresistible urge to live. Overcoming pain is the expression of our humanity.

About the Authors

MARIE-JOSÉE RIVARD

Marie-Josée Rivard holds a doctorate in health psychology from the Université du Québec in Montreal. Her dissertation, completed at the Montreal Heart Institute, dealt with the psychological issues faced by people with a heart problem. Now a clinical psychologist specializing in pain management, she has over eight years of experience in private practice. In 2000 she joined the Alan Edwards Pain Management Unit of the McGill University Health Centre at Montreal General Hospital.

As part of a multidisciplinary team of health professionals, she works with people of all ages who are living with pain; her main goal is the desire to help sufferers alleviate their pain. In this context, Dr. Rivard has supervised interns in psychology and residents in psychiatry and medicine, taught pain management at several Quebec universities, and lectured to public audiences and health care professionals.

Marie-Josée Rivard has been on the board of the Société québécoise de la douleur — the Quebec Pain Society — for several years and is currently president for 2013 to 2016. This organization brings together professionals from various fields who are interested in chronic pain; its mission is to encourage continuing education and promote interdisciplinary care for patients.

A member of the International Association for the Study of Pain (IASP), the Canadian Pain Society, and the Société québécoise d'hypnose (the Quebec Hypnosis Society), Dr. Rivard also sits on the education committee of the ACCORD program (Application concertée des connaissances et ressources en douleur),

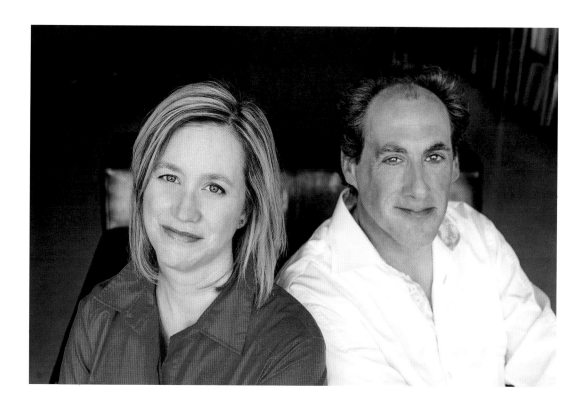

whose aim is to sensitize the public to chronic pain by explaining it and correcting misconceptions surrounding it. She has worked closely with others on several publications on various pain-related themes, and has hosted many discussions on pain management throughout Quebec.

DENIS GINGRAS

Denis Gingras has worked for several years on the borderline between science and literature, his two childhood passions. The holder of a doctorate in physiology from the Université de Montréal (1993) and a post-doctoral degree from McGill University (1996), for fifteen years he was a researcher specializing in oncology in the Hemato-oncology Service at Hôpital Sainte-Justine. During this time he collaborated with Dr. Richard Béliveau in writing *Foods that Fight Cancer* (Trécarré, 2005), inspired by their research into the anticancer potential of molecules found in plant-based foods. This became a genuine Quebec publishing phenomenon, translated into twenty-five languages, and it has caused a minor social revolution by sensitizing readers to the essential role eating habits and lifestyle habits play in preventing cancer and chronic illnesses in general. Since writing *Cooking with Foods That Fight Cancer* (2006) and *Eating Well, Living Well: An Everyday Guide for Optimum Health* (2008), Dr. Gingras has spent most of his professional time writing popular science books, notably *Death* (2010), published by Trécarré.

To Learn More ...

Chapter 1: The Problem of Pain

Melzack, R. "The Myth of Painless Childbirth." The John J. Bonica Lecture. *Pain* 19 (1984): 321–37.

Schopflocher, D., P. Taenzer, and R. Jovey. "The Prevalence of Chronic Pain in Canada." *Pain Research and Management* 16, no. 6 (2011): 445–50.

Boulanger, A., A.J. Clark, P. Squire, E. Cui, and G. Horbay. "Chronic Pain in Canada: Have We Improved Our Management of Chronic Noncancer Pain?" *Pain Research and Management* 12, no. 12 (2007): 39–47.

Ramage-Morin, L., and H. Gilmour. 2010. "Chronic Pain at Ages 12 to 44." *Statistics Canada, Health Reports* 21, no. 4 (2010): 1–9.

Gaumont, I. and S. Marchand. "La douleur est-elle sexiste? Mécanismes endogènes et hormones sexuelles." *Medicine/Sciences* 22 (2006): 1011–12.

Pain Proposal: Improving the Current and Future Management of Chronic Pain – A European Consensus Report. 2010.

Nguyen, C., S. Poiraudeau, M. Revel, and A. Papelard. "Lombalgie chronique: facteurs de passage à la chronicité." *Revue du Rhumatisme* 76 (2009): 537–42.

Public Health Agency of Canada. "Life with Arthritis in Canada: A Personal and Public Health Challenge." 2010.

Wolfe, F., D.J. Clauw, M. Fitzcharles, D.L. Goldenberg, R.S. Katz, P. Mease, A.S. Russel, I.J. Russell, J.B. Winfield, and M.B. Yunus. "The American College of Rheumatology Preliminary Diagnostic Criteria for Fibromyalgia and Measurement of Symptom Severity." *Arthritis Care & Research* 62, no. 5 (2010): 600–610.

Staud, R., J. Mease and D. A. Williams. "Expert Panel Supplement: Fibromyalgia Facts: Foundations for Assessment, Care, and Treatment Strategies." *The International Journal of Neuropsychiatric Medicine* 14, no. 12, suppl. 16 (2009).

Statistics Canada. *Canadian Community Health Survey: Public Use Microdata File.* 2007–2008.

Canadian Pain Coalition and the Canadian Pain Society/La Société Canadienne de la Douleur. 2011. *Pain in Canada Fact Sheet.* 2011.

Thomas, A. and R. Andrianne. "Douleur paroxistiques lombaires: la colique néphrétique." *Revue Médicale de Liège* 59, no. 4 (2004): 215–20.

International Association for the Study of Pain. *Global Year Against Headache: Trigemino-Autonomic Headaches.* 2011.

Fishman, Scott M., M.D., Jane C. Ballantyne, M.D., F.R.C.A., and James P. Rathmell, M.D., eds. *Bonica's Management of Pain.* 4th Edition. Philadelphia: Wolters Kluwer/Lippincott and Williams & Wilkins, 2010.

International Association for the Study of Pain. *Pain Clinical Updates: Diagnosis and Classification of Neuropathic Pain* 18, no. 7 (2010): 6.

Minor, J.S. and J.B. Epstein. "Burning Mouth Syndrome and Secondary Oral Burning." *Otolaryngologic Clinics of North America* 44 (2011): 205–19.

Luckhaupt, S, J.M. Dahlhamer, B.W. Ward, M.H. Sweeney, J.P. Sestito, and G.M. Calvert. "Prevalence and Work-Relatedness of Carpal Tunnel Syndrome in the Working Population, United States, 2010 National Health Interview Survey." *American Journal of Industrial Medicine* 4 (2012).

Schmader, K.E. "Epidemiology and Impact on Quality of Life of Postherpetic Neuralgia and Painful Diabetic Neuropathy." *The Clinical Journal of Pain* 18 (2002): 350–54.

Portenoy, R.K. "Treatment of Cancer Pain." *The Lancet* 377, no. 9784 (2011): 2236–47.

Elbert, T. "Pain from Brain: Can We Remodel Neural Circuitry That Generates Phantom Limb Pain and Other Forms of Neuropathic Pain?" *Neuroscience Letters* 507 (2012): 95–96.

International Association for the Study of Pain. *Global Year Against Headache: Tension-Type Headache.* 2011.

International Association for the Study of Pain. *Global Year Against Headache: Migraine.* 2011.

International Association for the Study of Pain. *Global Year Against Headache: Epidemiology of Headache.* 2011.

International Association for the Study of Pain. *Pain Clinical Updates: Visceral Pain* 13, no. 6 (2005).

Chapter 2: Pain under the Magnifying Glass

Beecher, H. "Pain in Men Wounded in Battle." *Annals of Surgery* 123, no. 1 (1946): 96–105.

Melzack, R. and P. Wall. "Pain Mechanisms: A New Theory." *Science* 150, no. 3699 (1965): 971–79.

H. Dehen. "Lexique de la douleur." *La Presse Médicale* 12 (1983): 1459–60. French translation of list of pain terms. International Association for the Study of Pain. Merskey et al. *Pain* 6 (1979): 249–52.

Marchand, S. *Le Phénomène de la douleur.* 2nd Edition. Montréal: Éditions Chenelière Éducation. 2009.

McGill University. "The Brain from Top to Bottom." http://thebrain.mcgill.ca/ (accessed March 31, 2012).

Kuner, R. Central Mechanism of Pathological Pain. *Nature Medicine* 16, no. 11 (2010): 1258–66.

Bar-On, E., D. Weigl, R. Parvari, K. Katz, R. Weitz, and T. Steinberg. "Congenital Insensitivity to Pain." *The Journal of Bone and Joint Surgery* 84-b, no. 2 (2002): 252–57.

Basbaum, A.I. and D. Julius. "Toward Better Pain Control." *Scientific American* (2006): 60-67.

Chapter 3: Lives turned upside down

Lautenbacher, S., B. Kundermann, and J.C. Krieg. "Sleep Deprivation and Pain Perception." *Sleep Medicine Reviews* 10 (2006): 357–69.

Lavigne, G., B.J. Sessle, M. Choinière, and P.J. Soja, eds. *Sleep and Pain.* Seattle: International Association for the Study of Pain Books, 2007.

Lavigne, G., A. Nashed, C. Manzini, and M.C. Carra. "Does Sleep Differ Among Patients With Common Musculoskeletal Pain Disorders?" *Current Rheumatological* Reports 13 (2011): 535–42.

Bell, R.F., J. Borzan, E. Kalso, and G. Simonnet. "Food, Pain and Drugs: Does it Matter What Pain Patients Eat?" In *Pain* (2012).

Chapter 4: When Emotions Enter the Picture

Roy, M., M. Piché, J.I. Chen, I. Peretz, and P. Rainville. "Cerebral and Spinal Modulation of Pain by Emotions." *Proceedings of the National Academy of the Sciences USA* 106, no. 49 (2009): 20900–05.

DSM-IV-TR. *Cas cliniques: manuel diagnostique et statistique des troubles mentaux.* (French version of *DSM-IV-TR Casebook: A Learning Companion to the Diagnostic and Statistical Manual of Mental Disorders*, published in 2002 by The American Psychiatric Association). Paris: Elsevier Masson, 2002.

Sullivan, M.J.L., S.R. Bishop, and J. Pivik. "The Pain Catastrophizing Scale: Development and Validation." *Psychological Assessment* 7, no. 4 (1995): 524–32.

Statistics Canada. *Canadian Community Health Survey.* 2000–2001.

Adams, H., T. Ellis, W.D. Stanish, and M.J.L. Sullivan. "Psychosocial Factors Related to Return to Work Following Rehabilitation of Whiplash Injury." *Journal of Occupational Rehabilitation* 17 (2007): 305–15.

Asmundson, G.J.G. and J. Katz. "Understanding the Co-Occurrence of Anxiety Disorders and Chronic Pain: A State of the Art." *Depression and Anxiety* 26 (2009): 888–901.

Trost, Z., K. Vangronsveld, S.J. Linton, J. Quartana, and M.J.L. Sullivan. "Cognitive Dimension of Anger in Chronic Pain." *Pain* 153 (2012): 515–17.

Beck, J.G. and J.D. Clapp. "A Different Kind of Comorbidity: Understanding Posttraumatic Stress Disorder and Chronic Pain." *Psychological Trauma: Theory, Research, Practice and Policy* 3, no. 2 (2011): 101–108.

Chapter 5: The Therapeutic Challenge: An Overview of Medical Treatments

"The Montreal Declaration: Access to Pain Management is a Fundamental Human Right." *Pain* 152 (2011): 2373–674.

Melzack, R. *Questionnaire ALGIE du Service de Psychologie de l'Hôtel-Dieu de Montréal.* Translation by F. Viguié of the *McGill Pain Questionnaire*, modified version (1983). In Melzack, R. and P. Wall. 1975. *Le Défi de la douleur.* 3rd Edition, 1989. Paris and Montréal: Edisem-Vigot/Chenelière and Stanké, 1984.

Chartrand, M.R., L. Courtois, J. Paré, and D. Richer, in collaboration with J.P. Dumas. *Vous avez de la douleur? Glace ou chaleur?* Montréal: Ordre professionnel de la physiothérapie du Québec, 2008.

Lussier, D., P. Beaulieu, F. Porreca, and A.H. Dickenson. *Pharmacology of Pain.* Seattle: International Association for the Study of Pain Press, 2010.

Chapter 6: Pain Self-Management

Rainville, P., G.H. Ducan, D.D. Price, B. Carrier, and C. Bushnell. "Pain Affect Encoded in Human Anterior Cingulate but not Somatosensory Cortex." *Science* 277 (1997): 968–71.

Faymonville, M.É., J. Joris, M. Lamy, P. Maquet, and S. Laureys. "Hypnose: des bases neurophysiologiques à la pratique clinique." *Conférences d'actualisation* (2005): 59–69.

Nicholas, M. "The Pain Self-Efficacy Questionnaire." *European Journal of Pain* 11 (2007): 153–63.

Morin, Charles M. *Vaincre les ennemis du sommeil.* Montréal: Éditions de l'Homme, 1997.

Bourassa, M., H. Golan, and C. Leclerc. *L'hypnose en médecine, médecine dentaire et en psychologie.* Montréal: Éditions Cursus Universitaire and Éditions du Méridien, 1999.

IMAGE CREDITS

CONTACT INFORMATION

Dr Marie-Josée Rivard
Alan Edwards Pain Management Unit

McGill University Health Centre
Montreal General Hospital, Office E19.128
1650 Cedar Avenue
Montreal, Québec
H3G 1A4

Telephone: 514-934-8222

Also in the Your Health Series

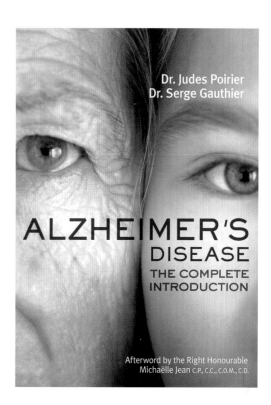

ALZHEIMER'S DISEASE
The Complete Introduction
By Dr. Judes Poirier and
Dr. Serge Gauthier

Alzheimer's disease is a reality in millions of lives and a serious concern for seniors and their loved ones. In developed countries where people are living longer than ever before, the incidence of Alzheimer's is reaching epidemic proportions, according to the World Health Organization. For families, sufferers, and caregivers, the need for reliable, clear, and concrete information has never been greater.

Alzheimer's Disease: The Complete Introduction is a comprehensive guide to the disease and its effects: getting a diagnosis, the ways it can progress and be managed, strategies for supporting sufferers and accessing care, legal concerns, and more. This guide addresses every aspect of the disease from the first doctor's visit to the long-term measures that can drastically improve the lives of sufferers and those close to them.

Diane B. Boivin M.D., Ph.D.
Foreword by Ève Van Cauter

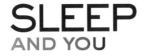

SLEEP
AND YOU
Sleep Better, Live Better

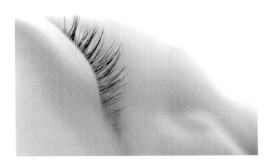

SLEEP AND YOU
Sleep Better, Feel Better
By Diane B. Boivin, M.D., Ph.D.

Why do we need to sleep? For those of who pass nights staring at the ceiling, the question is beside the point. In fact, we are all sleeping less, and worse, than ever. Despite this, we know that losing sleep or sleeping fitfully has consequences for our health and well being. What can we do when sleep just won't come?

In nine fascinating chapters, Dr. Diane B. Boivin lays out exactly why sleeping well is essential to good health. She explains, in a clear and accessible way, the phenomena associated with sleep: our individual sleep needs; circadian rhythms and problems linked to our biological clocks; the links between insomnia, stress, and obesity; why those suffering from anxiety or depression can have trouble sleeping; snoring; sleep apnea; night terrors; and dreams, among others. Special attention is given to sleep disturbances affecting night workers and new mothers.

An abundantly illustrated, practical guide for everyone trying to reclaim their sleep.

Coming in March 2015

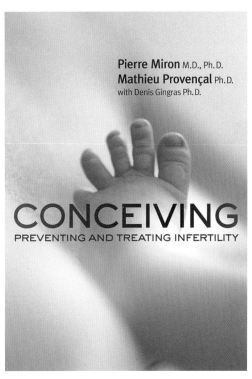

Conceiving
Preventing and Treating Infertility
By Dr. Pierre Miron, M.D., Ph.D.
and Mathieu Provençal, Ph.D.
with Denis Gingras, Ph.D.

In recent years, infertility has become a medical phenomenon that affects more and more adults of reproductive age. In western countries, between 10 and 15 percent of couples are infertile. These couples are victims of a silent human tragedy that can cause major suffering and significantly erode quality of life. This work presents a guide to reproductive difficulties and the medical approaches that can help prevent and treat infertility.

Available at your favourite bookseller

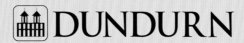

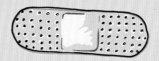

VISIT US AT
Dundurn.com
@dundurnpress
Facebook.com/dundurnpress
Pinterest.com/dundurnpress